GYMNASTICS

HOW TO BE THE BEST TEAMMATE

A Gymnast's Guide to Teamwork and Success

RITA BROWN

2 TIME OLYMPIC COACH

Rita Brown

RJC PUBLISHING

©2025 by Rita Brown
RJC Publishing
8443 Via Vittoria Way
Orlando, Florida 32819

ISBN: 978-1-938975-01-1
info@gymcert.com
www.gymcert.com

Copyright Notice

No part of this publication may be reproduced, stored in a retrieval system, or transmitted, in any form or by any means - electronic, mechanical, photocopying, recording, or otherwise - without the prior permission of RJC Publishing.

Disclaimer

This book is intended as a guide only. The publisher and author are not engaged in rendering legal, technical, or medical advice. For specific concerns, consult qualified professionals.

Every effort has been made to provide complete and accurate information on this subject. Readers are strongly advised to seek guidance and instruction from GymCert publications, USAG Safety Certified Coaches or Instructors, or Coaches with Risk Management Certifications through USA Gymnastics Organization.

The author and RJC Publishing shall have neither liability nor responsibility to any person or entity for any injury, loss, or damage caused directly or indirectly by the information contained in this book.

Design and Production

RJC Publising
Cover Design: Kurt Merkel / Rita Brown
Photos: Rita Brown / ChatGPT / XGrok
Printed in the United States
All rights reserved under U.S. and International copyright laws.

DEDICATION

This book is dedicated to five extraordinary gymnasts who not only achieved the pinnacle of athletic excellence by becoming Olympians but also exemplified what it means to be great teammates, competitors, and role models for gymnasts around the world:

- **1988 Olympian Brandy Johnson**
- **1992 Olympian Wendy Bruce**
- **1996 Olympian Eileen Diaz (Puerto Rico)**
- **2004 Olympian Carly Patterson**
- **2004 Olympian Mohini Bhardwaj**

Your dedication, passion, and unwavering spirit continue to inspire the gymnastics community and beyond. Thank you for setting the bar high and showing that true greatness lies not only in accomplishments but also in character.

Rita Brown

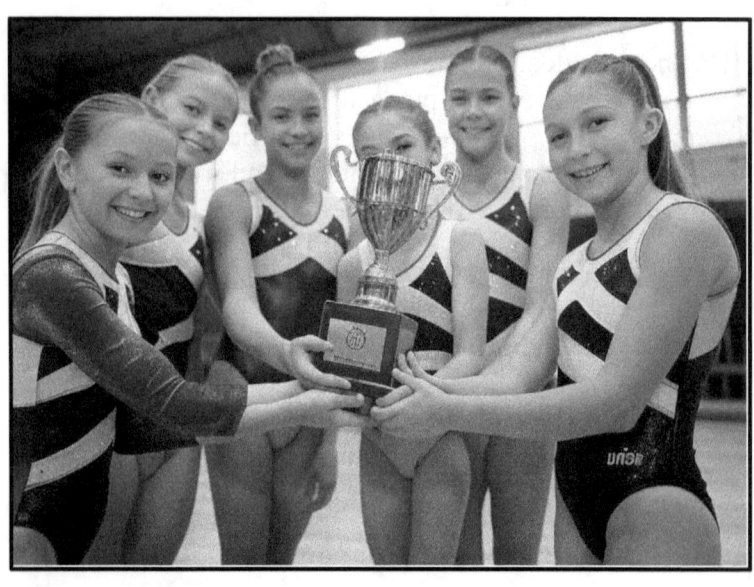

FORWARD:

Gymnastics is more than a sport of individual skill and talent - it's a discipline that thrives on teamwork and collaboration. Success in gymnastics is not achieved alone; it requires the collective effort of a supportive and unified team. This book explores the essential qualities that make a great teammate and provides practical guidance on how to develop them.

Throughout these pages, we'll dive into the importance of communication, respect, responsibility, trust, support, work ethic, mental toughness, and goal setting. By embracing and embodying these values, you can elevate not only your own performance but also contribute to the success of your entire team. Together, let's unlock the potential to achieve greatness both in the gym and beyond.

Rita Brown

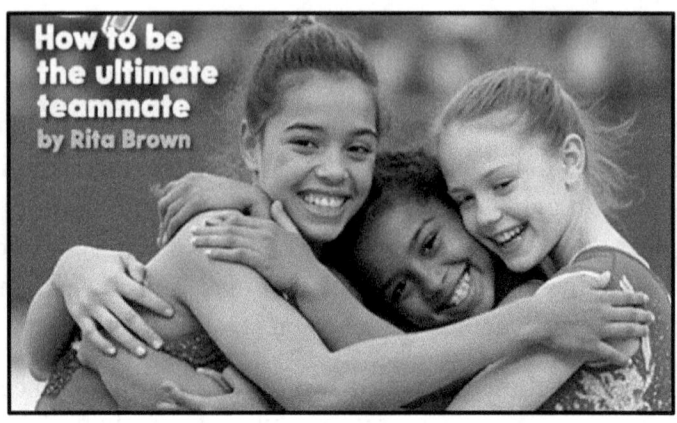

INTRODUCTION

GYMNASTICS: How to Be the Best Teammate Ever

Welcome to the world of gymnastics, where strength meets grace, and individual talent combines with teamwork to create something truly extraordinary. This book is your guide to understanding how to be the best teammate - both on and off the mat.

My name is Rita Brown, and I've had the honor of coaching Olympic-level gymnasts. Over the years, I've learned that gymnastics isn't just about mastering flips and routines - it's also about building trust, supporting one another, and growing together as a team.

Whether you're new to gymnastics or already a seasoned athlete, this book is here to inspire and guide you. Together, we'll explore what makes a team stronger, how to handle challenges, and how to celebrate victories as one. So, let's get started and discover what it takes to become the ultimate teammate!

Rita Brown
Two-time Olympic Gymnastics Coach

Rita Brown

TABLE OF CONTENTS

Dedication 3
Forward 5
Introduction 7
What is Gymnastics? 11
The Importance of Teamwork in Gymnastics 12

Chapter 1: Understanding the Ultimate Teammate 14
Chapter 2: Becoming a Role Model 19
Chapter 3: Building Trust Within Your Team 22
Chapter 4: Handling Challenges as a Team 27
Chapter 5: Celebrating Successes as a Team 31
Chapter 6: Embracing Commitment 36
Chapter 7: Passion 41
Chapter 8: The Art of Goal Setting 47
Chapter 9: Overcoming Obstacles 53
Chapter 10: The Power of Support 59
Chapter 11: The Power of Teamwork in Gymnastics 65
Chapter 12: Being a Good Listener 69
Chapter 13: Sportsmanship 74
Chapter 14: Navigating Disappointment 78
Chapter 15: Staying Motivated Throughout the Season. .. 83
Chapter 16: Building Leadership Skills 87
Chapter 17: Being Prepared for Practice 91
Chapter 18: Responsibilities Beyond Training 96
Conclusion: 100
Let's Journal 103
About The Author 107
Note Pages 110

Rita Brown

WHAT IS GYMNASTICS?

Gymnastics is an amazing sport that challenges both your body and mind. It's about performing skills like flips, tumbles, and balancing acts with strength and precision. Whether you're flipping on a beam, swinging on bars, or jumping high on a trampoline, gymnastics is all about combining effort and skill.

Did you know there are different types of gymnastics? Here are some examples:

- **Artistic Gymnastics**: This is the most popular type and includes events like the vault, uneven bars, balance beam and floor exercise for girls, and floor exercise, pommel horse, rings, vault, parallel bars and horizontal bar for boys.

- **Rhythmic Gymnastics**: This style involves performing with hoops, balls, clubs, ribbon and ropes in graceful routines.

- **Trampoline Gymnastics**: Athletes perform high-flying routines on trampolines.

- **Acrobatic Gymnastics**: This type involves working with a partner or group to create stunning stunts and formations.

Gymnastics isn't just about competing. It's also about teamwork. When you support your teammates and work together, the whole team gets stronger. Throughout this book, you will learn how to grow as a teammate and contribute to your team's success. Gymnastics might seem like an individual sport, but being part of a team is just as important. When gymnasts work together, they build trust, improve communication, and create a supportive environment where everyone can thrive.

The Importance of Team Work

Why is teamwork important? Let's break it down:

- **Building Trust**: Imagine a teammate spotting you during a tricky skill. Trusting them makes you feel safe and helps you perform better.

- **Communicating Well**: Good communication is key. Whether you're giving advice, asking for help, or just cheering someone on, your words can make a big difference.

- **Supporting Each Other**: A great teammate knows how to lift others up. Whether it's celebrating a win or helping a teammate through a tough moment, support keeps the team strong.

GYMNASTICS: How To Be the Best Teammate

Here are some tips to improve teamwork:

1. **Be a Good Listener**: Pay attention when your teammates or coach are talking. Ask questions if you don't understand something.

2. **Use Kind Words**: Always encourage your teammates and avoid negative comments.

3. **Celebrate Together**: Cheer for your team during competitions and share in each other's successes.

Try This: Think of one thing you can do today to make your teammate feel appreciated. Maybe it is giving them a compliment or helping them with a skill they're working on.

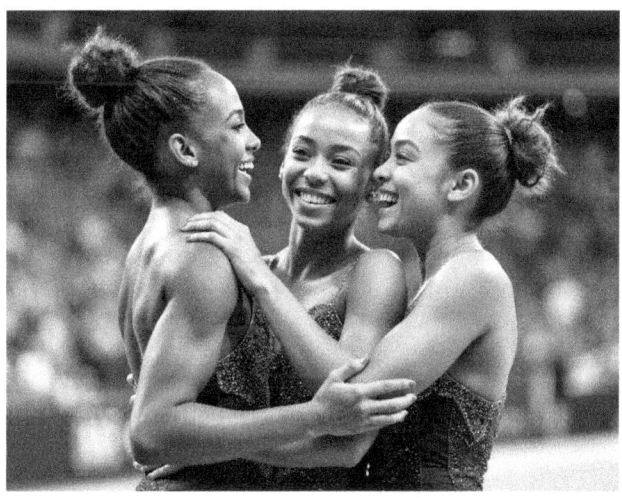

Chapter 1:

Understanding the Ultimate Teammate

Welcome to the exciting world of gymnastics, where strength, grace, and teamwork come together to create unforgettable moments. As gymnasts, coaches, and teammates, we know that success in this sport isn't just about individual talent - it's about the collective effort of a team working as one.

But what does it mean to be an "ultimate teammate"? Let's break it down.

Embracing Your Role

Every member of a gymnastics team plays a unique role. Some gymnasts are incredible at flips, while others excel at balance or flexibility. Some might be the motivators—always ready with a cheer or a high five. Whatever your strengths, it's important to embrace your role and give it your all.

Think of your team as a puzzle. Each gymnast is a piece, and the team isn't complete without everyone playing their part. Ask yourself: What can I bring to the team? How can I make my team stronger?

GYMNASTICS: How To Be the Best Teammate

What Makes an Ultimate Teammate?

Here are some qualities that define an ultimate teammate:

1. **Dependability**: Show up to practice on time, be prepared, and give 100% effort every time. Your team needs to know they can count on you.

2. **Encouragement**: Be the cheerleader your teammates need. Whether someone nails a skill or struggles with a routine, your words can make a big difference.

3. **Respect**: Treat your teammates, coaches, and even competitors with kindness and understanding. Respect builds trust and strong relationships.

4. **Resilience**: Challenges and setbacks are part of gymnastics. The ultimate teammate doesn't give up. They keep trying and inspire others to do the same.

Creating a Positive Environment

Great teammates lift each other up. When you create a positive environment, everyone feels supported and motivated. Here's how:

- **Celebrate Successes**: Big or small, every achievement deserves recognition. Cheer the loudest for your teammates when they succeed.

- **Encourage Growth**: If someone is struggling, they offer to help or give them advice. Show that you're there for them.

- **Avoid Negativity**: Gossip and criticism have no place in a supportive team. Focus on building each other up instead.

Teammate Spotlight

Here's an inspiring story of teamwork in action:

During a recent competition, one gymnast on a team twisted her ankle during warm-ups. Instead of letting the setback discourage them, her teammates rallied around her. They adjusted their routines, cheered extra loudly from the sidelines, and supported her throughout the day. The team didn't just perform well - they left the competition feeling closer and stronger than ever.

Tips for Being the Best Teammate

Here are some practical ways to become the ultimate teammate:

1. **Communicate Openly**: Share your thoughts and listen to others. Good communication is the foundation of teamwork.

GYMNASTICS: How To Be the Best Teammate

2. **Be Reliable**: Always follow through on your commitments, whether it's showing up to practice or helping a teammate.

3. **Set a Good Example**: Your actions can inspire others. Show dedication, focus, and a positive attitude every day.

4. **Show Gratitude**: Thank your teammates and coaches for their support. A simple "thank you" goes a long way.

Try This Activity

Take a moment to think about your team. Write down three things you love about being part of it and one way you can contribute even more. Share your ideas with a teammate or coach. This simple exercise can strengthen your bond and inspire everyone to work together even better.

Being an ultimate teammate isn't just about what happens in the gym. It's about how you treat others, how you handle challenges, and how you lift up the people around you. By embracing your role, creating a positive environment, and always striving to do your best, you can become the kind of teammate every gymnast dreams of having.

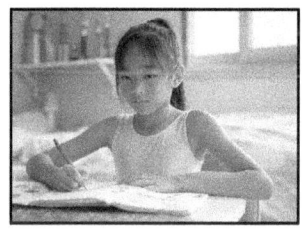

Rita Brown

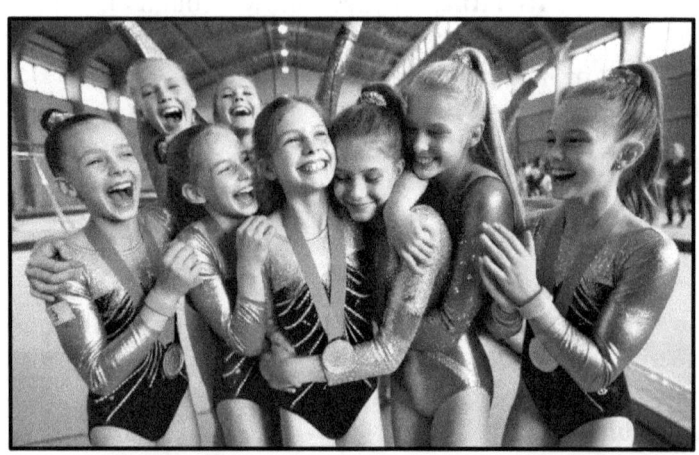

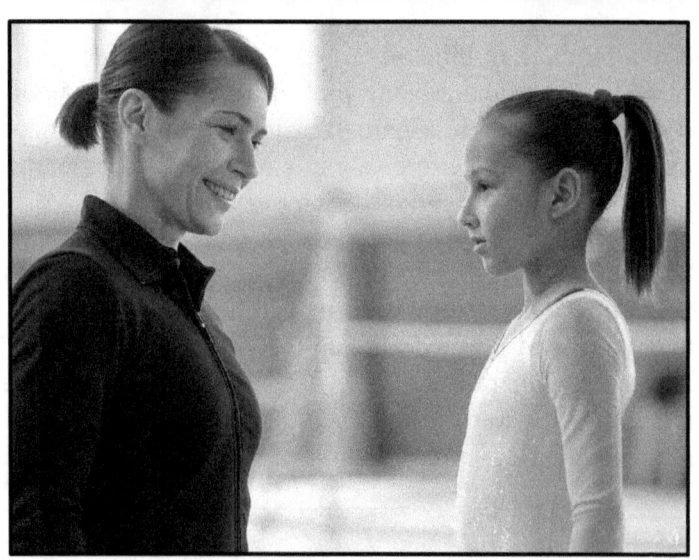

Chapter 2:
Becoming a Role Model

Being a role model isn't about being perfect—it's about striving to be your best and inspiring others along the way. In gymnastics, role models lead by example, show kindness, and lift others up. Whether you're the team captain or a beginner, you have the power to be someone others look up to.

Why Role Models Matter

Role models set the tone for the entire team. When you work hard, stay positive, and treat others with respect, your teammates are more likely to do the same. A team full of role models is a team that supports each other and achieves great things.

Think about someone you admire. What do they do that inspires you? Chances are, they're dedicated, kind, and resilient. These are qualities you can develop in yourself to become a role model for others.

How to Be a Role Model

Here are some ways to lead by example and inspire your teammates:

1. **Work Hard**: Put your best effort into every practice and routine. Hard work is contagious, and your dedication will motivate others.

2. **Stay Positive**: Even when things are tough, focus on what you can do to improve. A positive attitude helps your team stay motivated.

3. **Be Kind**: Offer help to teammates who are struggling and celebrate their successes. Small acts of kindness go a long way.

4. **Handle Challenges Gracefully**: Everyone faces setbacks, but role models show resilience. Instead of getting discouraged, they find ways to overcome obstacles and learn from them.

The Ripple Effect

Being a role model doesn't just affect you - it has a ripple effect on your entire team. When you show dedication and kindness, others are inspired to do the same. This creates a positive team culture where everyone feels supported and motivated to do their best.

Real-Life Role Model: Simone Biles

Simone Biles is one of the greatest gymnasts of all time, but she's also an incredible role model. She's known for her

GYMNASTICS: How To Be the Best Teammate

hard work, humility, and support for her teammates. Even during tough moments, Simone has shown resilience and grace, inspiring gymnasts around the world to strive for greatness.

Activity: Reflect on Your Role

Think about how you can be a role model for your team. Write down:

- One way you already inspire your teammates.

- One area where you can improve to set an even better example.

Share your thoughts with a teammate or coach and encourage them to do the same. Together, you can build a team full of role models.

Being a role model isn't about being the best gymnast - it's about being the best teammate. When you lead by example, you inspire others to work hard, stay positive, and support each other. By becoming a role model, you help your team grow stronger and achieve more together.

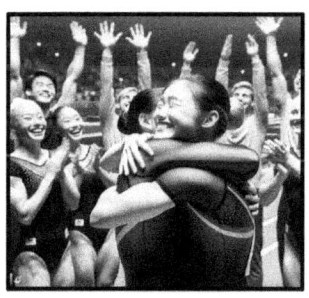

Chapter 3:
Building Trust Within Your Team

Trust is the foundation of any great team. Without it, teammates can't rely on each other, and the team's performance suffers. In gymnastics, where safety and teamwork are essential, building trust is even more important.

Why Trust Matters

Imagine you're practicing a new skill on the uneven bars, and your teammate is spotting you. Would you feel confident if you didn't trust them? Trust allows gymnasts to take risks, push their limits, and support one another through challenges.

When trust is strong, teams:

- Communicate openly and honestly.
- Work together more effectively.
- Feel safe and supported, both emotionally and physically.

How to Build Trust

Building trust doesn't happen overnight, but small actions every day can make a big difference. Here are some ways to create a foundation for trust within your team:

1. **Be Honest**: If you make a mistake, own up to it. Honesty shows your teammates that you're reliable and accountable.

2. **Follow Through on Promises**: If you say you'll do something, make sure you do it. Consistency builds trust over time.

3. **Be Supportive**: Celebrate your teammates' successes and encourage them when they're struggling. Show that you have their back.

4. **Respect Boundaries**: Everyone has different comfort levels. Respecting those boundaries shows your teammates that you value their feelings.

The Role of Communication

Clear and open communication is a key part of building trust. Here's how to improve your communication skills:

- **Listen Actively**: Pay attention when your teammates or coach are speaking. Nod, ask questions, and show that you're engaged.

- **Speak Honestly but Kindly**: Share your thoughts but always do so in a respectful way. For example, instead of saying, "You messed up," try, "Let's work on this together."

- **Check In Regularly**: Ask your teammates how they're feeling and if they need help. Regular check-ins show that you care.

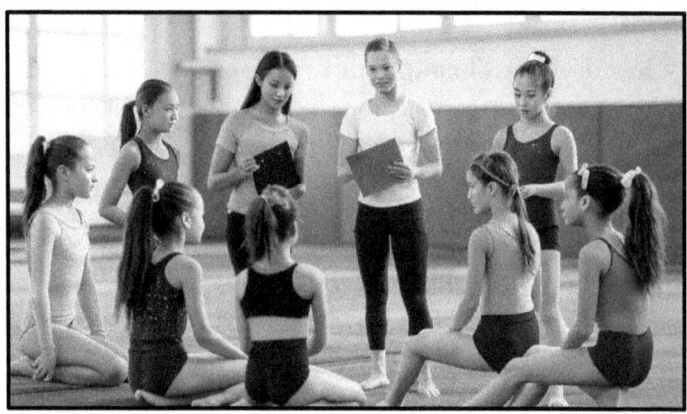

Trust-Building Activities

Here are some fun activities to help your team build trust:

1. **Partner Spotting Practice**: Pair up with a teammate and practice spotting each other during a simple skill. This builds trust in your physical safety.

GYMNASTICS: How To Be the Best Teammate

2. **Team Challenges**: Work together to complete a group challenge, like creating a synchronized routine or solving a puzzle.

3. **Compliment Circle**: Sit in a circle and have each person share one positive thing about the teammate next to them. This activity helps build emotional trust and connection.

Overcoming Challenges to Trust:

Sometimes, trust can be broken - whether it's due to a misunderstanding, mistake, or conflict. Here's how to rebuild trust:

1. **Acknowledge the Issue**: Talk openly about what happened and how it affected the team.

2. **Apologize and Forgive**: If you made a mistake, apologize sincerely. If someone else made a mistake, be willing to forgive and move forward.

3. **Set Clear Expectations**: Agree on how to avoid similar issues in the future and commit to those actions.

Activity: Trust Reflection

Think about a time when you felt truly supported by a teammate. What did they do to earn your trust? Write it down and share it with them as a thank-you. Then, think about one way you can strengthen trust within your team and put it into action.

Building trust isn't always easy, but it's worth the effort. When trust is strong, your team will feel more connected, confident, and capable of achieving great things together.

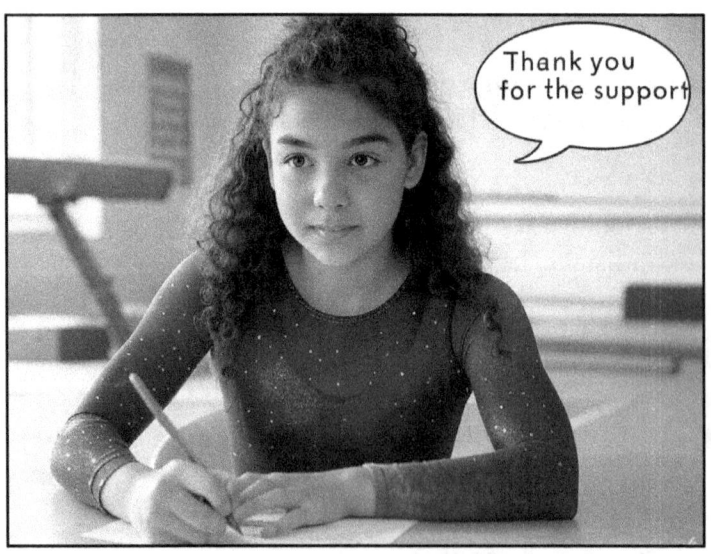

Chapter 4:
Handling Challenges as a Team

In gymnastics, as in life, challenges are inevitable. Whether it's a tough practice, a missed routine, or a disagreement among teammates, overcoming obstacles is part of the journey. How your team handles challenges can make or break your success.

Why Challenges Are Important

Challenges might feel frustrating in the moment, but they're also opportunities to grow stronger as a team. When you face a problem together, you learn to communicate, adapt, and support one another. These skills don't just make you a better team - they make you better gymnasts and individuals.

Think of challenges as stepping stones. Each one you overcome brings your team closer and prepares you for even greater achievements.

Common Challenges Teams Face

Some of the most common challenges gymnastics teams encounter include:

1. **Performance Pressure**: Competitions can be stressful, and the pressure to perform well can weigh on everyone.

2. **Injuries**: When a teammate gets hurt, it affects the entire team emotionally and physically.

3. **Miscommunication**: Misunderstandings can lead to frustration and conflict if not addressed.

4. **Setbacks in Practice**: Struggling with a routine or skill can test everyone's patience and morale.

How to Overcome Challenges

Here are some strategies your team can use to tackle challenges head-on:

1. **Stay Positive**: Focus on what you can learn from the situation instead of dwelling on what went wrong.

2. **Work Together**: Brainstorm solutions as a team. When everyone contributes, you'll find better answers faster.

3. **Support Each Other**: Remind your teammates that you're in this together. A little encouragement goes a long way.

4. **Talk It Out**: If conflict arises, address it calmly and respectfully. Clear communication can resolve most issues.

Real-Life Example: Turning Setbacks into Success

At a recent competition, a team faced a major setback when their top gymnast fell during her floor routine. Instead of letting it ruin their day, the team rallied around her. They reminded her of her strengths, cheered louder than ever, and nailed their remaining routines. In the end, they placed second - a victory they achieved together.

Activity: Challenge Plan

Think about a challenge your team is currently facing. Write down:

- What the challenge is?
- Why it's important to overcome it?
- One action you can take to help your team handle it.

Share your plan with your teammates and encourage them to create their own plans. Working together, you can tackle any obstacle.

The Power of Resilience

Resilience is the ability to bounce back from difficulties. It's one of the most important qualities a team can have. By staying resilient, you show that no challenge is too big to overcome.

Remember: Every challenge is an opportunity to grow. When you face it as a team, you come out stronger, closer, and ready to take on whatever comes next.

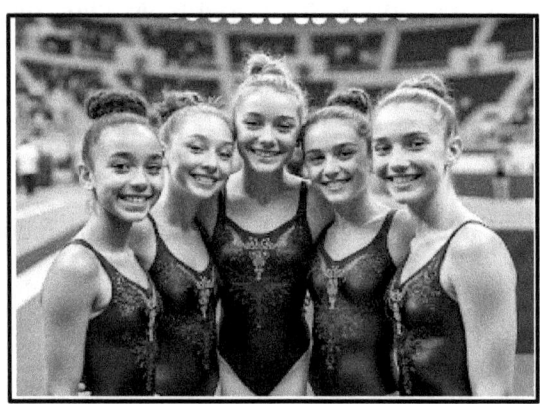

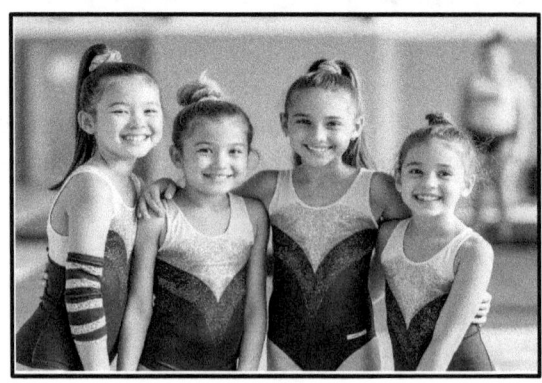

Chapter 5:

Celebrating Successes as a Team

Success in gymnastics comes in many forms. It might be nailing a difficult routine, achieving a personal best, or simply overcoming a tough practice. While individual accomplishments are worth celebrating, team successes bring everyone together and remind us why being part of a team is so special.

The Importance of Celebrating Success

Celebrating success is not just about having fun - it's about building morale, strengthening bonds, and motivating each other to keep striving for greatness. When you take the time to recognize achievements, you show your teammates that their hard work matters.

Think of celebrations as a way to recharge your team's energy. Whether it's cheering loudly after a great performance or organizing a team outing, these moments create memories that fuel your team's spirit.

Different Types of Success to Celebrate

Here are some examples of successes that deserve recognition:

1. **Competition Wins**: Placing in a meet or achieving a high score is always worth celebrating.

2. **Personal Bests**: When a teammate improves their performance, it's a victory for the whole team.

3. **Overcoming Challenges**: Did someone master a tricky skill or bounce back after a tough day? That's worth cheering for.

4. **Teamwork Moments**: Celebrate times when the team worked well together, whether it was during practice, a performance, or supporting each other.

How to Celebrate as a Team

Celebrations don't have to be elaborate. Sometimes, the simplest gestures mean the most. Here are some ideas for celebrating successes:

1. **Cheer Each Other On**: During practices or competitions, cheer loudly for your teammates. Your enthusiasm can boost their confidence.

2. **Team Huddles**: After a big moment, gather the team for a group cheer or pep talk. It's a great way to share the excitement.

3. **Compliments and High Fives**: Recognize individual efforts with a kind word, a pat on the back, or a high five.

4. **Celebrate Milestones**: Mark special occasions, like achieving a season goal or overcoming a major obstacle, with a team dinner or outing.

5. **Create Traditions**: Develop fun team rituals, like a special cheer or handshake, to celebrate victories.

Balancing Celebration and Focus

While celebrating is important, it's also essential to stay grounded and focused on future goals. Here's how to strike a balance:

- **Acknowledge Effort**: Celebrate the hard work that led to success, not just the outcome. This keeps the team motivated to continue improving.

- **Keep It Short and Sweet**: Enjoy the moment, but don't lose sight of what's ahead. Use celebrations as a way to refocus and energize the team.

- **Learn From Success**: Reflect on what went well and how you can build on it. Successes are opportunities for growth, just like challenges.

Real-Life Example: A Winning Tradition

One gymnastics team created a "Victory Jar" where they wrote down successes - big and small - on slips of paper. At the end of each season, they gathered to read the notes and relive their favorite moments. This simple tradition helped them appreciate their progress and strengthened their bond as a team.

Activity: Celebrate Your Team

Take a moment to recognize your team's recent successes. Write down:

- A specific achievement you're proud of.

- How the team contributed to that success.

- One way you can celebrate together.

Share your ideas with your teammates and plan a celebration that reflects your team's unique personality.

Celebrating success isn't just about enjoying the moment. It's about building a culture of positivity, gratitude, and motivation. When your team takes the time to appreciate each other's efforts, you create an environment where everyone feels valued and inspired to reach new heights.

GYMNASTICS: How To Be the Best Teammate

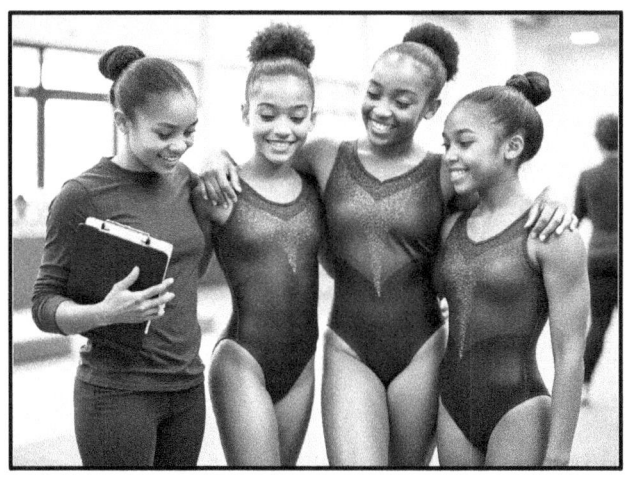

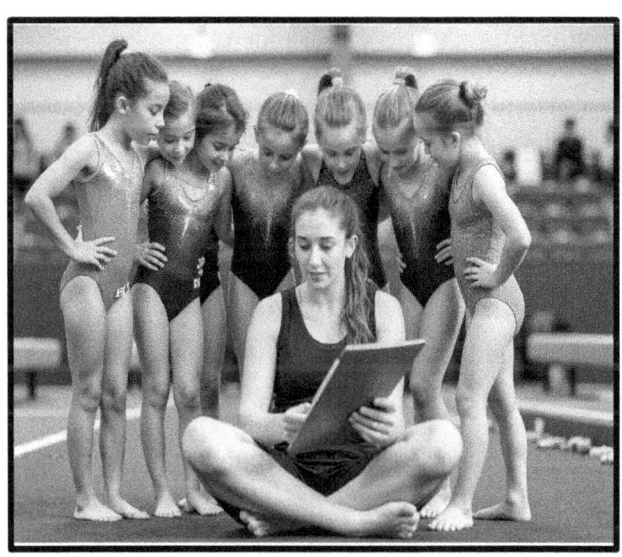

Chapter 6:
Embracing Commitment

Commitment is the backbone of any successful gymnastics team. It's what keeps you showing up to practice, striving for improvement, and supporting your teammates no matter what. But commitment isn't just about hard work, it's about staying dedicated to your goals and your team, even when things get tough.

What Does Commitment Look Like?

Commitment shows up in many ways during your gymnastics journey. Here are some examples:

1. **Attendance**: Being present at every practice and event, ready to give your best effort.

2. **Preparation**: Coming to practice with the right mindset and tools, like proper attire, water, and a focus on learning.

3. **Consistency**: Putting in the effort every day, not just when it's convenient or easy.

4. **Team Support**: Encouraging your teammates and being there for them during highs and lows.

GYMNASTICS: How To Be the Best Teammate

Why Commitment Matters

Commitment isn't just about you; it's about how your actions affect the entire team. When everyone is committed, the team becomes stronger, more cohesive, and better prepared for success. Commitment also helps you build trust with your teammates and coaches, showing them that you're reliable and dedicated.

How to Strengthen Your Commitment

If you want to deepen your commitment to gymnastics, try these strategies:

1. **Set Clear Goals**: Write down what you want to achieve in gymnastics, both individually and as part of your team. Keep these goals in mind as you practice.

2. **Stay Focused**: Block out distractions during practice and competitions. Remember why you're there and what you're working towards.

3. **Find Motivation**: On tough days, remind yourself of your love for gymnastics and the progress you've made so far.

4. **Hold Yourself Accountable**: Take responsibility for your actions, whether it's showing up on time, or giving your best effort.

Balancing Commitment and Flexibility

While commitment is essential, it's also important to stay flexible. Life can throw unexpected challenges your way, and learning to adapt without losing sight of your goals is a valuable skill. For example:

- If you miss a practice, communicate with your coach and make a plan to catch up.

- If you're struggling with a skill, stay committed to improving while being patient with yourself.

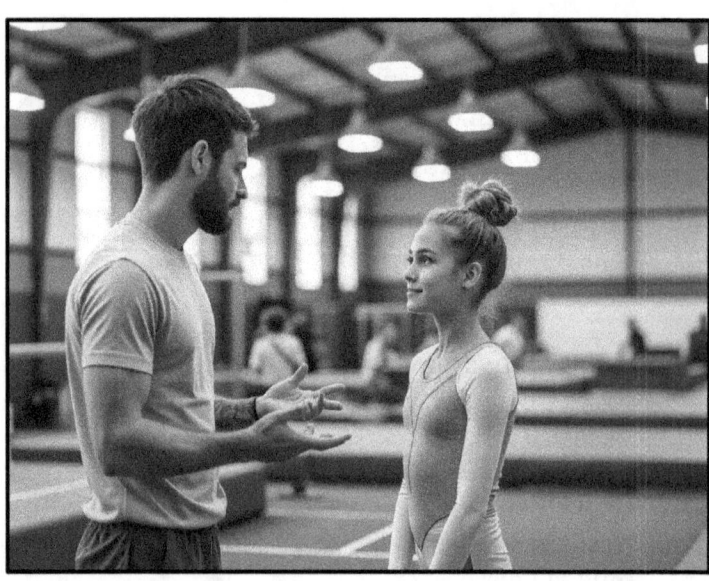

Real-Life Example: The Power of Perseverance

A young gymnast named Mia struggled with her balance beam routine for weeks. Instead of giving up, she stayed committed to practicing every day. Her teammates cheered her on, and her coach provided guidance. Eventually, Mia nailed her routine at a competition, proving that commitment and perseverance pay off.

Activity: Commitment Tracker

Create a commitment tracker to help you stay focused on your goals. Include:

- Daily practice habits (e.g., stretching, conditioning).
- Weekly progress on skills you're working on.
- A section for reflecting on your accomplishments.

Review your tracker regularly to celebrate your dedication and identify areas for improvement.

Commitment is about showing up, giving your best effort, and staying true to your goals. When you embrace commitment, you not only grow as a gymnast but also inspire your teammates to do the same. Together, your dedication will lead to incredible achievements.

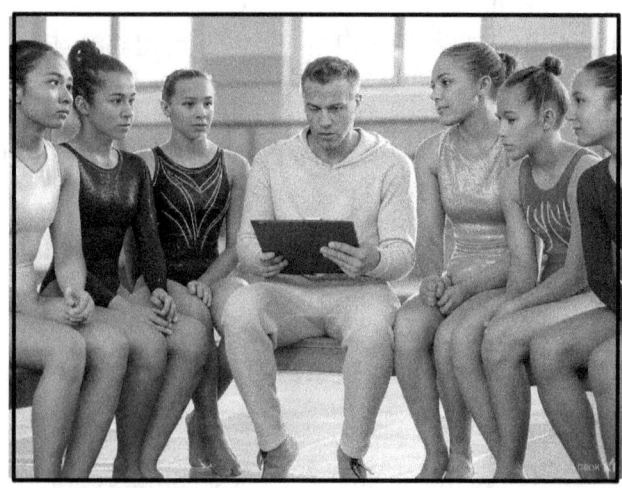

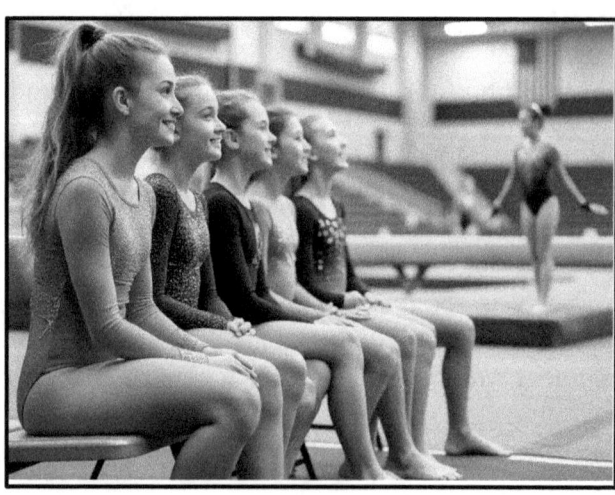

Chapter 7:
Passion: Fueling Your Gymnastics Journey

Passion is the spark that ignites your journey in gymnastics. It's what keeps you coming back to practice, dreaming of new skills, and pushing through tough days. Without passion, the hard work and dedication required in this sport can feel overwhelming. But with passion, every challenge becomes an opportunity to grow and achieve.

What Is Passion in Gymnastics?

Passion in gymnastics isn't just about loving the sport—it's about finding joy in the process and staying motivated to improve. Passion is what makes the hours of practice, the sore muscles, and the setbacks all worth it.

Passion might look like:

1. **Excitement for Practice**: Looking forward to each session and enjoying the chance to learn.

2. **Curiosity to Improve**: Always wanting to try new skills and perfect existing ones.

3. **Pride in Progress**: Feeling accomplished with each small victory, whether it's mastering a routine or building strength.

Why Passion Matters

Passion is more than just a feeling - it's a powerful motivator. Here's why it matters:

1. **Sustains Dedication**: Passion helps you stay committed, even on difficult days.

2. **Builds Resilience**: When you truly love what you're doing, it's easier to bounce back from setbacks.

3. **Inspires Others**: Passion is contagious. When your teammates see your enthusiasm, it can inspire them to give their best, too.

How to Cultivate Passion

Not every day in gymnastics will feel exciting, but there are ways to keep your passion alive:

1. **Focus on What You Love**: Think about the aspects of gymnastics that bring you joy. Is it the feeling of flying through the air, the satisfaction of nailing a skill, or the friendships you've built?

2. **Set Fun Goals**: In addition to competitive goals, set personal ones that excite you, like mastering a move you've always admired.

3. **Celebrate Small Wins**: Recognize and appreciate the progress you're making, even if it's just a little improvement each day.

4. **Mix It Up**: If practice feels routine, try something new, like working on a different apparatus or creating a fun mini routine.

Overcoming Passion Burnout

Even the most passionate gymnasts can feel burnt out at times. Here's how to reignite your love for the sport:

- **Take a Break**: Sometimes stepping away for a day or two can help you return refreshed and ready to go.

- **Reflect on Your Why**: Remember why you started gymnastics and what you've accomplished so far.

- **Find Inspiration**: Watch videos of your favorite gymnasts or attend a competition to remind yourself of what's possible.

- **Talk to Your Team**: Share how you're feeling with teammates or coaches. Their encouragement can help you rediscover your spark.

Real-Life Example: Rekindling Passion

Sophia loved gymnastics but felt discouraged after struggling with a new skill. Instead of giving up, she took a moment to reflect on why she started. She remembered the thrill of her first meet and the pride she felt in her progress. With encouragement from her coach and teammates,

Sophia regained her enthusiasm and approached practice with renewed energy.

Activity: Passion Journal

Create a passion journal to help you stay connected to what you love about gymnastics. Include:

- A list of reasons why you love gymnastics.
- Your favorite memories from practice, competitions, or team events.
- A space to write about your feelings after practice, focusing on what went well.

Review your journal whenever you need a reminder of why gymnastics is important to you.

GYMNASTICS: How To Be the Best Teammate

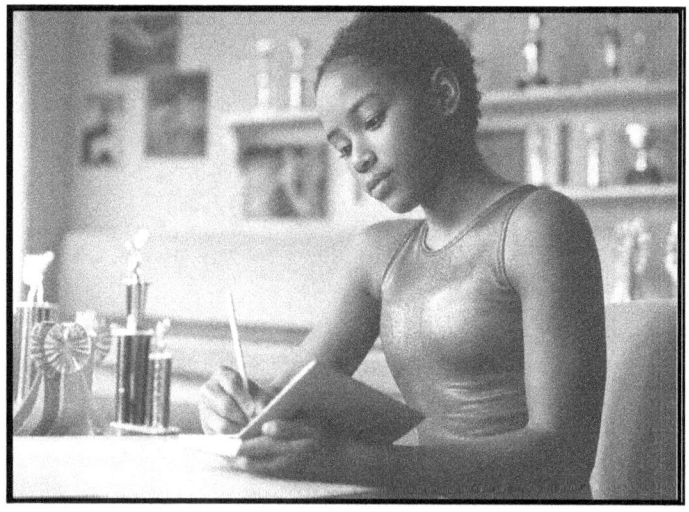

Passion is the heart of your gymnastics journey. It's what keeps you motivated, helps you overcome challenges, and inspires those around you. By staying connected to what you love about the sport, you can fuel your journey and achieve amazing things, both as an individual and as part of your team.

Rita Brown

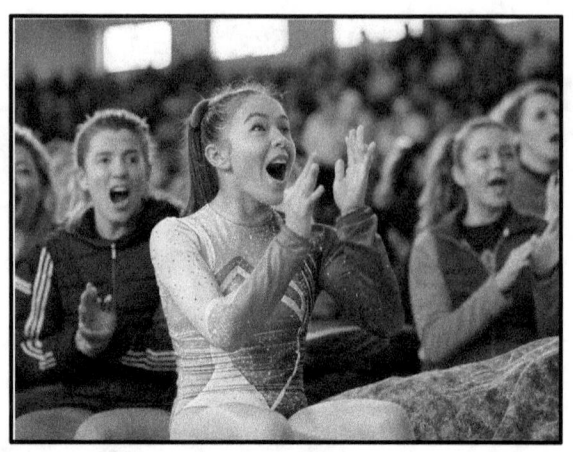

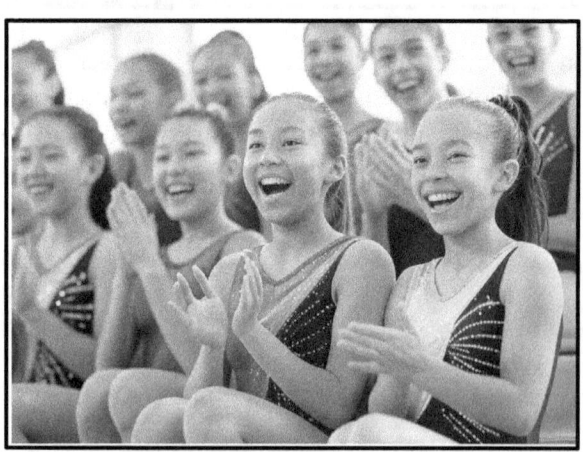

Chapter 8:
The Art of Goal Setting

Goals are the roadmap to success in gymnastics. They give you direction, purpose, and motivation to keep pushing forward. Whether you're dreaming of mastering a new skill, winning a competition, or simply improving your strength, setting goals can help you stay focused and make steady progress.

Why Set Goals?

Setting goals helps you:

1. **Stay Focused**: With clear goals, you know exactly what you're working toward.

2. **Measure Progress**: Goals let you track how far you've come and celebrate milestones along the way.

3. **Build Confidence**: Achieving goals, no matter how small, boosts your self-esteem and shows you what you're capable of.

4. **Stay Motivated**: Goals give you a reason to keep going, even when practice gets tough.

Types of Gymnastics Goals

It's important to set a variety of goals to challenge yourself and keep things exciting. Here are three types of goals to consider:

1. **Short-Term Goals**: These are things you can achieve in a few weeks or months, like perfecting a specific move or improving flexibility.

2. **Long-Term Goals**: These take more time and effort, such as competing at a higher level or mastering advanced skills.

3. **Team Goals**: Work with your teammates to set goals that benefit the entire team, like improving teamwork during routines or achieving a group score at a meet.

How to Set Effective Goals

Use the SMART method to create goals that are:

- **Specific**: Clearly define what you want to achieve (e.g., "Improve my balance beam routine").

- **Measurable**: Make it easy to track your progress (e.g., "Land my dismount 10 times in a row").

- **Achievable**: Set goals that are challenging but realistic (e.g., "Add one new skill to my routine this month").

GYMNASTICS: How To Be the Best Teammate

- **Relevant**: Focus on goals that align with your overall gymnastics journey (e.g., "Strengthen core muscles to improve stability").

- **Time-Bound**: Give yourself a deadline to stay motivated (e.g., "Achieve this by the end of the season").

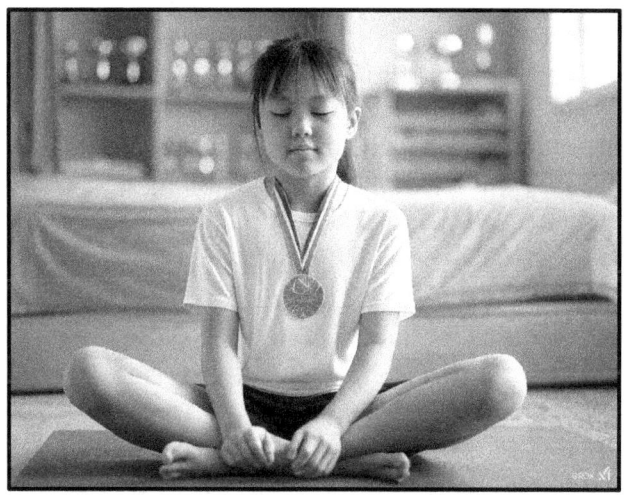

Visualize Your Goals

Overcoming Goal-Setting Challenges

Sometimes, setting and sticking to goals can feel overwhelming. Here's how to tackle common challenges:

1. **Break It Down**: Divide big goals into smaller, manageable steps.

2. **Stay Flexible**: Be willing to adjust your goals if needed. Progress isn't always linear, and that's okay.

3. **Celebrate Effort**: Even if you don't achieve a goal right away, recognize the hard work you've put in.

Real-Life Example: Reaching for the Stars

Ethan, a young gymnast, set a goal to master a back tuck within three months. He broke the goal into smaller steps: strengthening his legs, practicing drills, and working with his coach for feedback. By staying focused and committed, Ethan achieved his goal and felt a huge sense of accomplishment.

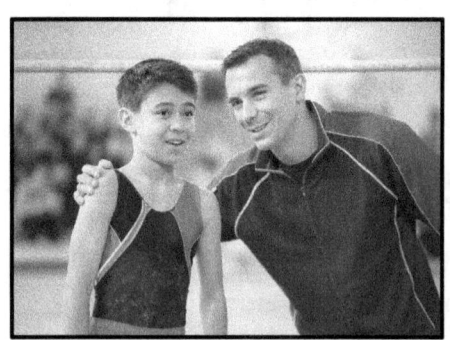

Activity: Goal Setting Map

Create a goal-setting map to visualize your progress. Include:

- Your ultimate gymnastics goal.

GYMNASTICS: How To Be the Best Teammate

- Three short-term goals that will help you get there.
- Action steps for each short-term goal.

Review your map regularly and adjust it as needed. Celebrate each milestone you reach to stay motivated.

Setting goals is an essential part of growth in gymnastics. By defining what you want to achieve and working toward it step by step, you can turn your dreams into reality and inspire others to do the same.

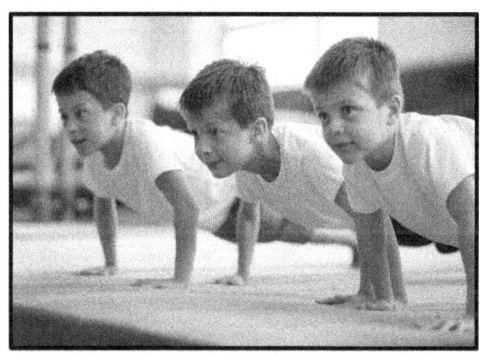

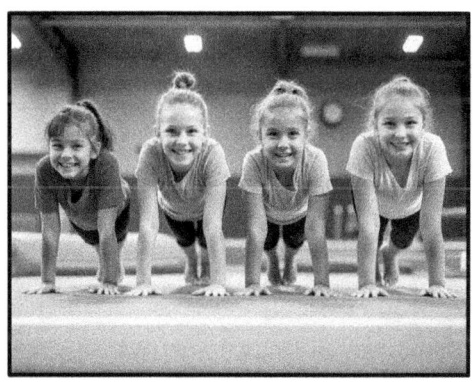

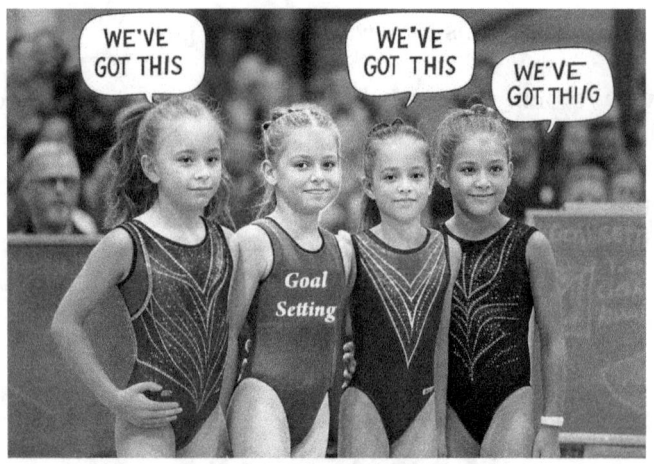

Team Goal Setting "Unity"

Chapter 9:
Overcoming Obstacles

Obstacles are a natural part of every gymnast's journey. Whether it's a challenging skill, a tough competition, or an unexpected setback, learning how to overcome obstacles is a critical skill that will serve you both on and off the mat. Facing these challenges with resilience and determination is what sets great gymnasts apart.

Why Obstacles Matter

Obstacles might seem frustrating in the moment, but they're essential for growth. Each challenge you face is an opportunity to learn, improve, and build the mental toughness that gymnastics requires. Overcoming obstacles not only makes you a better gymnast but also teaches you life skills like perseverance, problem-solving, and adaptability.

Think of obstacles as stepping stones that help you reach your full potential. Without them, there'd be no opportunity to rise above and achieve greatness.

Common Obstacles Gymnasts Face

Here are some challenges gymnasts often encounter and tips for tackling them:

1. **Fear of New Skills**: Trying a difficult or unfamiliar move can be intimidating.

    - **Tip**: Break the skill into smaller steps and practice each part until you feel confident.

    - **Example**: If you're learning a back handspring, start with drills like backbends and bridge kickovers.

2. **Performance Anxiety**: Competing in front of judges and a crowd can be nerve-wracking.

    - **Tip**: Focus on your preparation and visualize yourself succeeding. Deep breathing can also help calm nerves.

3. **Setbacks in Practice**: Struggling with a routine or failing to master a skill can be discouraging.

    - **Tip**: Remember that progress isn't always linear. Celebrate small improvements and trust the process.

4. **Injuries**: Physical setbacks can be frustrating and require patience.

    - **Tip**: Follow your coach's and doctor's advice for recovery. Use the time to focus on mental preparation or flexibility exercises.

Mindset Matters

Your mindset plays a huge role in how you handle obstacles. Adopting a positive and growth-oriented attitude can make all the difference. Here's how to cultivate the right mindset:

- **Embrace Challenges**: Instead of seeing obstacles as roadblocks, view them as opportunities to grow.

- **Stay Patient**: Progress takes time, and setbacks are normal.

- **Focus on What You Can Control**: While you can't control every challenge, you can control your effort and attitude.

Strategies for Overcoming Obstacles

Here are practical strategies to help you overcome any challenge:

1. **Break It Down**: Divide big challenges into smaller, manageable tasks.

2. **Seek Support**: Lean on your teammates, coaches, and family for encouragement and advice.

3. **Visualize Success**: Picture yourself overcoming the obstacle and achieving your goal.

4. **Stay Consistent**: Keep showing up and putting in the effort, even when progress feels slow.

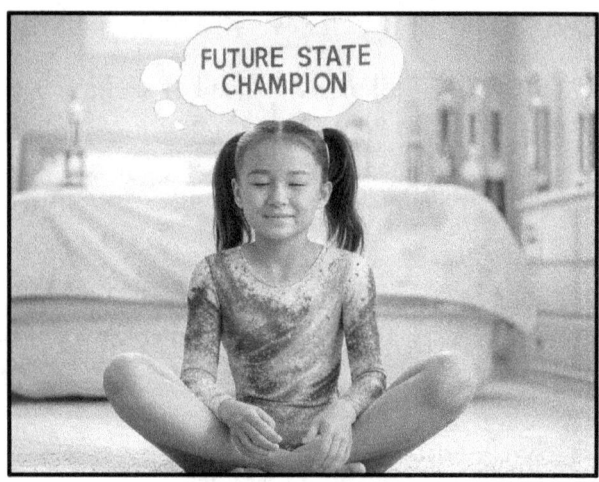

Visualize Success

Real-Life Example: Conquering the Balance Beam

Lila struggled with her confidence on the balance beam after a fall during practice. Instead of giving up, she worked with her coach to rebuild her trust in the apparatus. They started with simple exercises and gradually increased difficulty. With patience and determination, Lila regained her confidence and performed a flawless routine at her next competition.

GYMNASTICS: How To Be the Best Teammate

Activity: Obstacle Reflection

Think about a recent obstacle you faced in gymnastics. Write down:

1. What the challenge was.

2. How you approached it.

3. What you learned from the experience.

Share your reflection with a teammate or coach. Discussing your challenges can provide new perspectives and inspire others.

The Power of Resilience

Resilience is your ability to bounce back from difficulties. By facing obstacles head-on and refusing to give up, you develop the strength and confidence to handle anything that comes your way. Remember: Every gymnast faces challenges, but it's how you respond that defines your journey.

Overcoming obstacles isn't just about gymnastics - it's about building the skills and mindset that will help you succeed in all areas of life. Embrace the challenges, and you'll discover how strong and capable you truly are.

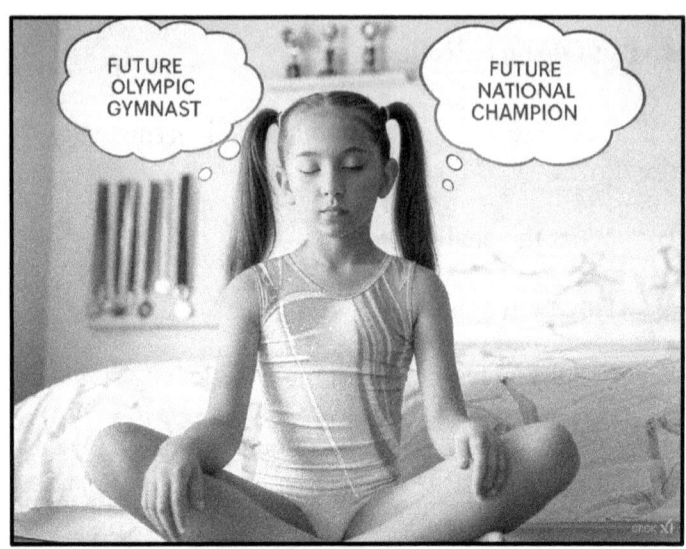

Keep Visualizing Your Dreams

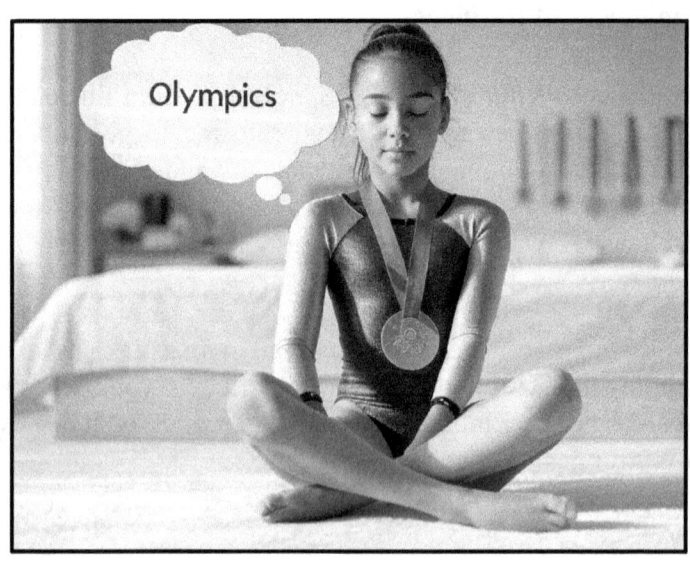

Chapter 10:
The Power of Support

Support is the glue that holds a gymnastics team together. Whether it's cheering for a teammate, offering a helping hand, or simply listening when someone needs to talk, support is what transforms a group of individuals into a family. By giving and receiving support, your team becomes stronger, more connected, and better equipped to achieve great things.

Why Support Matters

Support is essential because:

1. **It Builds Confidence**: Knowing that your teammates have your back gives you the courage to take risks and try new things.

2. **It Creates a Positive Environment**: When everyone feels supported, practices and competitions become more enjoyable and productive.

3. **It Strengthens Bonds**: Acts of support build trust and deepen relationships, helping your team work as one.

Ways to Support Your Teammates

Support comes in many forms. Here are some simple but powerful ways to show up for your team:

1. **Cheer Loudly**: During practice or competitions, cheer for your teammates. Your encouragement can boost their confidence and energy.

2. **Be a Spotter**: Help your teammates feel safe by spotting them during challenging skills.

3. **Offer Help**: If you see someone struggling with a skill, offer to practice with them or share tips that have worked for you.

4. **Celebrate Successes**: Acknowledge your teammates 'achievements, big or small, and share in their excitement.

5. **Be a Good Listener**: Sometimes, support is as simple as listening when a teammate wants to share their thoughts or feelings.

How to Ask for Support

It's okay to need help, and asking for support shows strength, not weakness. Here's how to ask for help when you need it:

GYMNASTICS: How To Be the Best Teammate

1. **Be Honest**: Let your teammates or coach know what you're struggling with and how they can help.

2. **Be Specific**: Explain exactly what you need, whether it's advice, a spot, or just someone to talk to.

3. **Be Grateful**: Thank your teammates for their support and let them know it means a lot to you.

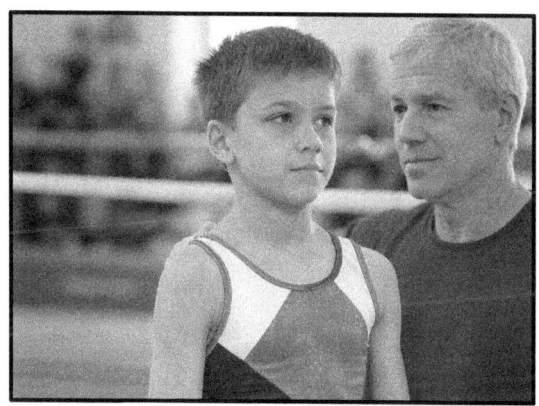

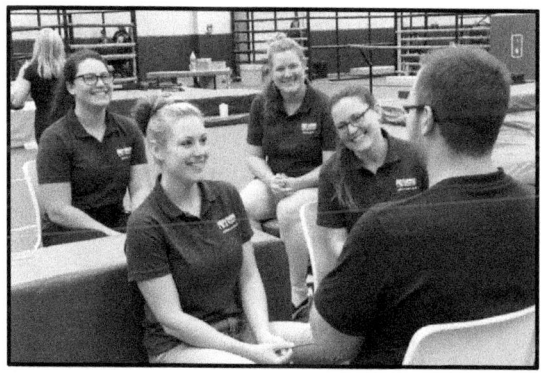

Coaches are always available for Support

Creating a Culture of Support

Support isn't just about individual acts—it's about creating a team culture where everyone feels valued and cared for. Here's how to foster a supportive environment:

- **Lead by Example**: Show your teammates what support looks like by offering encouragement and help whenever you can.

- **Encourage Inclusion**: Make sure everyone on the team feels welcome and included no matter their skill level or experience.

- **Address Conflicts Respectfully**: If disagreements arise, handle them calmly and respectfully to maintain a positive atmosphere.

Real-Life Example: A Team That Lifted Each Other Up

At a regional competition, one gymnast had a rough start to her floor routine. Instead of focusing on their own events, her teammates gathered at the sidelines, cheering her on with everything they had. Their encouragement helped her regain her confidence and finish strong. The team's unity and support inspired everyone at the meet.

GYMNASTICS: How To Be the Best Teammate

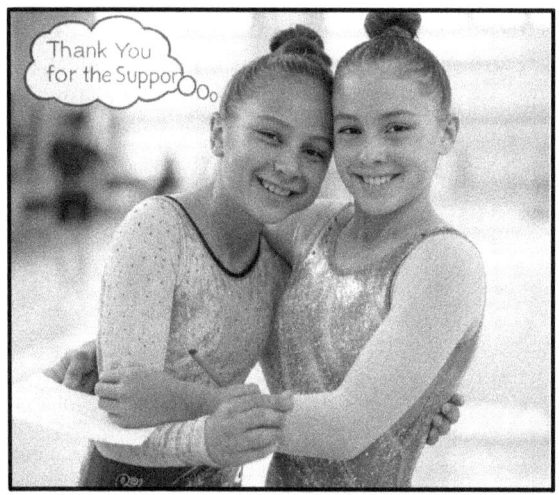

Activity: Support Circle

Create a support circle with your team. Sit in a circle and take turns sharing one thing you appreciate about the teammate to your left. This activity helps build trust, positivity, and connection among teammates.

The Ripple Effect of Support

Support has a ripple effect. When you lift up a teammate, they're more likely to pass that support on to someone else. Over time, these acts of kindness create a team culture where everyone feels valued, motivated, and ready to achieve their best.

By prioritizing support, you help your team grow stronger and closer, one act of kindness at a time. Together, you can accomplish more than you ever thought possible.

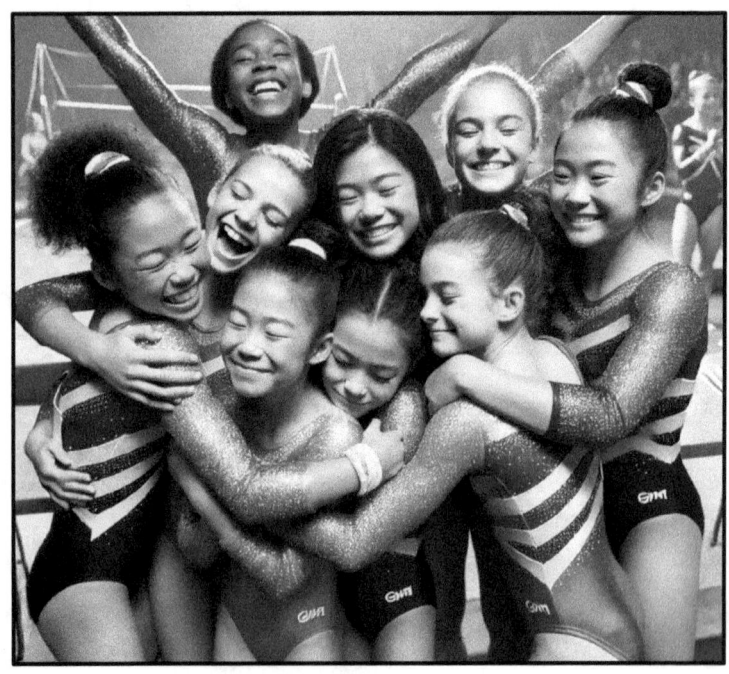

"We all win when we support each other."

Chapter 11:
The Dynamic Power of Teamwork in Gymnastics

Teamwork is at the heart of every great gymnastics team. While gymnastics often highlights individual routines, it's the collective effort and spirit of the team that truly drives success. Teamwork doesn't just happen naturally - it's something that must be cultivated and practiced every day.

Why Teamwork Matters

Teamwork is essential because:

1. **It Brings Out the Best in Everyone**: Working together allows teammates to push each other to achieve more than they could alone.

2. **It Builds Trust**: Relying on your teammates and supporting them in return creates a bond that strengthens the entire team.

3. **It Promotes Unity**: When everyone is working toward the same goal, the team feels more connected and focused.

Key Elements of Effective Teamwork

Here are the building blocks of strong teamwork:

1. **Communication**: Open and honest communication ensures that everyone is on the same page and working together effectively.

2. **Respect**: Valuing each teammate's contributions fosters a positive and collaborative environment.

3. **Shared Goals**: Aligning on team objectives helps everyone stay focused and motivated.

4. **Adaptability**: Being flexible and willing to adjust for the good of the team ensures smooth collaboration.

How to Foster Teamwork

To create a culture of teamwork, follow these strategies:

1. **Practice Together**: Use team drills and activities to build trust and coordination.

2. **Encourage Collaboration**: Assign tasks or routines that require teammates to work together and rely on each other.

3. **Celebrate Team Achievements**: Highlight moments of great teamwork during practices and competitions.

4. **Resolve Conflicts Quickly**: Address disagreements calmly and respectfully to keep the team united.

Real-Life Example: A Unified Team

A gymnastics team preparing for nationals realized that their strongest chance of success was by combining their individual strengths into a seamless team routine. They spent weeks practicing together, encouraging each other, and perfecting their timing. When the competition day arrived, their unity shone through, earning them top marks for teamwork and performance.

Activity: Teamwork Challenge

Organize a fun teamwork challenge during practice, such as creating a synchronized routine or working together to solve a gymnastics-themed puzzle. This activity will help your team build trust and learn how to rely on each other.

The Power of Teamwork

Teamwork is about more than just working together - it's about creating a sense of belonging, trust, and unity that pushes everyone to be their best. When your team prioritizes teamwork, you'll not only perform better but also create lasting memories and bonds that extend beyond gymnastics. Together, your team can achieve greatness.

Rita Brown

Chapter 12:
Being a Good Listener

Listening is one of the most powerful skills a teammate can have. It's the foundation of effective communication, trust, and understanding within a team. By becoming a good listener, you show your teammates that you value their thoughts, feelings, and perspectives, helping to create a supportive and harmonious team environment.

Why Listening Matters

Good listening is essential because:

1. **It Builds Trust**: When teammates feel heard, they're more likely to trust and rely on each other.

2. **It Strengthens Relationships**: Listening helps you connect with your teammates on a deeper level.

3. **It Prevents Misunderstandings**: Paying attention ensures that everyone is on the same page, reducing conflicts and confusion.

4. **It Promotes Collaboration**: Teams that listen to each other work more effectively toward shared goals.

How to Be a Good Listener

Listening is a skill that takes practice and intention. Here are some ways to improve your listening abilities:

1. **Focus on the Speaker**: Give your full attention to the person speaking. Make eye contact, nod, and avoid distractions like your phone or other conversations.

2. **Listen Without Interrupting**: Let your teammate finish their thoughts before responding. Interruptions can make them feel unheard.

3. **Ask Questions**: Show that you're engaged by asking clarifying questions or encouraging them to elaborate.

4. **Use Positive Body Language**: Lean slightly forward, smile, and maintain an open posture to show that you're actively listening.

5. **Summarize What You Hear**: Repeat back or paraphrase what your teammate says to confirm your understanding.

The Impact of Active Listening

Active listening goes beyond just hearing words, it involves understanding the speaker's emotions and intentions. Here's how it can positively impact your team:

- **Improves Communication**: Clearer understanding of ideas and feedback.

- **Resolves Conflicts**: Helps teammates feel heard and respected during disagreements.

- **Fosters Empathy**: Encourages you to see things from your teammate's perspective.

Real-Life Example: Listening in Action

During a practice session, one gymnast was feeling overwhelmed about an upcoming competition. Instead of dismissing her concerns, her teammate took the time to listen and ask questions about how she was feeling. The simple act of listening made her feel supported, and together they worked through strategies to ease her nerves. Their bond grew stronger, and the entire team benefited from their mutual support.

Activity: Listening Exercise

Try this activity to practice your listening skills:

1. Pair up with a teammate and take turns sharing a thought or concern.

2. The listener's goal is to focus entirely on the speaker, without interrupting or judging.

3. After the speaker finishes, the listener summarizes what they heard and asks one follow-up question.

Discuss how it felt to be truly listened to and how it can improve team communication.

Listening in Team Settings

Good listening doesn't just happen one-on-one. It's essential during team discussions and meetings. Here's how to listen effectively in group settings:

1. **Give Everyone a Chance to Speak**: Ensure that quieter teammates have the opportunity to share their thoughts.

2. **Avoid Side Conversations**: Stay focused on the person speaking and avoid distractions.

3. **Acknowledge Contributions**: Show appreciation for your teammates 'ideas, even if you don't agree with them.

The Rewards of Listening

When you prioritize listening, your team becomes more connected, understanding, and effective. Teammates who feel heard are more likely to communicate openly, collaborate willingly, and contribute their best efforts. By being a good listener, you strengthen your role as a teammate and help create a positive environment where everyone can thrive.

GYMNASTICS: How To Be the Best Teammate

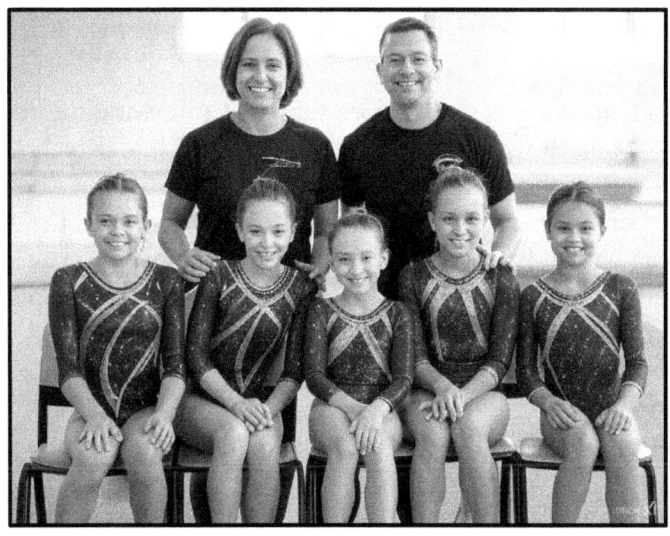

Listening is more than just hearing words; it's about making others feel valued and respected. By mastering this skill, you will enhance not only your own relationships but also the strength and unity of your entire team.

Chapter 13:

Sportsmanship: Humility and Respect in Action

Sportsmanship is about more than just following the rules - it's about showing humility, respect, and integrity both in and out of the gym. As a gymnast, your actions reflect not only on yourself but also on your team, coach, and the sport as a whole. By practicing good sportsmanship, you set a positive example and help create an environment where everyone can thrive.

What Is Sportsmanship?

Sportsmanship means treating others - teammates, competitors, coaches, and judges—with kindness and respect, regardless of the outcome. It's about celebrating success with humility and handling disappointment with grace.

Key aspects of sportsmanship include:

1. **Respect for Others**: Recognizing the efforts of teammates, competitors, and officials.

2. **Honesty**: Competing fairly and following the rules.

3. **Gratitude**: Appreciating the hard work of coaches, teammates, and event organizers.

4. **Grace Under Pressure**: Staying composed and respectful, even in challenging situations.

GYMNASTICS: How To Be the Best Teammate

Why Sportsmanship Matters

Good sportsmanship benefits everyone:

- **Builds Stronger Teams**: Respectful and supportive teammates create a positive team dynamic.

- **Earns Respect**: Competitors and coaches admire athletes who display humility and fairness.

- **Enhances the Sport**: When everyone upholds the values of sportsmanship, gymnastics becomes more enjoyable and inspiring for all.

How to Show Sportsmanship

Practicing good sportsmanship is simple but impactful. Here's how you can demonstrate it:

1. **Congratulate Competitors**: Whether you win or lose, take the time to acknowledge your opponents' efforts with a handshake or kind words.

2. **Support Your Teammates**: Celebrate their successes and encourage them during challenges.

3. **Respect Judges and Coaches**: Accept scores and feedback gracefully, even if you disagree.

4. **Avoid Negative Comments**: Speak positively about others and focus on uplifting your team.

Handling Wins and Losses with Grace

How you handle both victories and defeats says a lot about your character. Here are some tips:

- **After a Win**: Celebrate with humility. Recognize the efforts of your teammates and competitors who helped make the competition memorable.

- **After a Loss**: Reflect on what you learned and how you can improve. Congratulate the winners and use the experience as motivation to grow.

Real-Life Example: A True Champion

At a national competition, a gymnast named Ava won the gold medal in her division. Instead of focusing solely on her victory, she took the time to congratulate each of her competitors and thank the judges. Her humility and kindness made a lasting impression and showed everyone what it means to be a true champion.

Activity: Sportsmanship in Action

Try this exercise with your team:

1. After your next practice or competition, take a moment to reflect on how you showed sportsmanship.

GYMNASTICS: How To Be the Best Teammate

2. Write down one example of how you supported a teammate, competitor, or coach.

3. Share your reflections with the team and discuss how sportsmanship made a difference in the experience.

The Long-Term Impact of Sportsmanship

Sportsmanship isn't just about what happens in the gym, it's a mindset that carries over into all areas of life. By treating others with respect, staying humble, and leading with integrity, you set the stage for success both as a gymnast and as a person.

Remember: Medals and trophies may fade, but the impression you leave through your actions lasts forever. Be the teammate, competitor, and person who others admire for your character, and you'll make a lasting impact on your team and the sport of gymnastics.

Chapter 14:
Navigating Disappointment and Failure

Disappointment and failure are inevitable in gymnastics, just as they are in life. Whether it's missing a routine, falling short of a personal goal, or facing a tough competition result, these moments can feel disheartening. But they're also opportunities to grow stronger, learn valuable lessons, and build resilience. By navigating disappointment with a positive mindset, you can turn setbacks into steppingstones toward success.

Understanding Disappointment and Failure

Disappointment happens when our expectations don't align with reality. Failure often feels like a dead end, but it's actually a chance to reevaluate and improve. Remember, even the most accomplished gymnasts have faced setbacks - and it's their ability to persevere that sets them apart.

Why Facing Failure is Important

Failure is not the opposite of success; it's part of the journey. Here's why it matters:

1. **Teaches Resilience**: Bouncing back from failure builds mental toughness and determination.

2. **Encourages Growth**: Setbacks push you to identify weaknesses and work on them.

3. **Builds Empathy**: Experiencing failure helps you understand and support teammates when they face challenges.

4. **Shapes Perspective**: Learning to see failure as a steppingstone rather than a roadblock helps you stay motivated.

How to Navigate Disappointment

When disappointment strikes, these strategies can help you move forward:

1. **Acknowledge Your Feelings**: It's okay to feel upset or frustrated. Allow yourself to process your emotions instead of bottling them up.

2. **Reflect on the Experience**: Ask yourself what went wrong and what you can learn from it. Reflection turns mistakes into opportunities for growth.

3. **Talk to Someone You Trust**: Share your feelings with a teammate, coach, or family member. They can offer support and perspective.

4. **Focus on Improvement**: Identify specific steps you can take to do better next time. Create a plan and commit to it.

Turning Failure Into Motivation

Instead of letting failure hold you back, use it as fuel to propel yourself forward. Here's how:

- **Set New Goals**: Use what you learned from the setback to create fresh, achievable objectives.

- **Stay Positive**: Remind yourself of past successes and how you overcame challenges before.

- **Celebrate Effort**: Recognize the hard work you put in, even if the outcome wasn't what you hoped for.

Real-Life Example: Bouncing Back

During a regional meet, a gymnast named Ethan fell twice during his pommel horse routine, costing his team valuable points. While he initially felt devastated, his coach encouraged him to focus on what he could control: his preparation and mindset. Ethan spent the next month refining his routine and building his confidence. At the next competition, he delivered a nearly flawless performance, helping his team secure a top spot.

Activity: Reframe Your Setbacks

Try this exercise to shift your perspective on failure:

1. Write down a recent disappointment or failure.

2. List three things you learned from the experience.

3. Identify one positive outcome that came from facing the challenge.

Share your insights with a teammate or coach and discuss how you can support each other in navigating setbacks.

Supporting Teammates Through Disappointment

When a teammate faces disappointment, your support can make a big difference. Here's how to help:

- **Offer Encouragement**: Remind them of their strengths and past successes.

- **Listen Without Judging**: Let them share their feelings without interrupting or offering unsolicited advice.

- **Help Them Reframe**: Encourage them to see the setback as a temporary challenge, not a permanent failure.

The Resilience Advantage

Learning to navigate disappointment and failure isn't just a gymnastics skill - it's a life skill. By facing challenges head-on and refusing to give up, you build the resilience needed to achieve your goals and inspire those around you.

Remember: Every champion has faced setbacks. What defines them isn't how they fell but how they got back up. Embrace disappointment as part of your journey, and you'll come out stronger, more determined, and ready for whatever comes next.

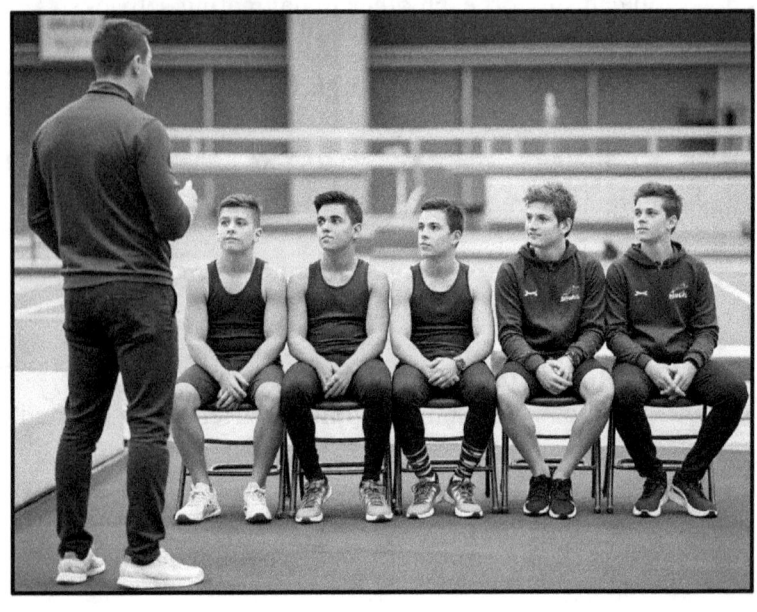

The coach and teammates support each other.

Chapter 15:
Staying Motivated Throughout the Season

Staying motivated in gymnastics isn't always easy. Between long practices, tough competitions, and the ups and downs of the season, even the most dedicated athletes can feel their enthusiasm waver. However, maintaining motivation is key to achieving your goals and supporting your team. By finding ways to stay inspired, you can keep pushing forward and make the most of every moment in the gym.

Why Motivation Matters

Motivation is what drives you to work hard, overcome obstacles, and keep striving for excellence. It helps you:

1. **Stay Focused**: Motivation keeps your eyes on the prize, even when distractions arise.

2. **Push Through Challenges**: When things get tough, your motivation reminds you why you started.

3. **Support Your Team**: A motivated gymnast inspires others, creating a positive and driven team culture.

Sources of Motivation

Motivation can come from many places. Here are some sources to tap into throughout the season:

1. **Personal Goals**: Focus on what you want to achieve, whether it's mastering a new skill or improving your performance.

2. **Team Goals**: Remember that your efforts contribute to the success of the entire team.

3. **Passion for Gymnastics**: Reflect on why you love the sport and the joy it brings you.

4. **Encouragement from Others**: Let the support of your teammates, coaches, and family fuel your determination.

How to Stay Motivated

Here are strategies to maintain your motivation throughout the season:

1. **Celebrate Progress**: Take time to acknowledge your improvements, no matter how small. Progress is a powerful motivator.

2. **Set Short-Term Goals**: Break the season into smaller milestones to keep things manageable and rewarding.

3. **Visualize Success**: Picture yourself achieving your goals and how it will feel when you get there.

4. **Mix Up Your Routine**: Avoid burnout by adding variety to your practices, such as trying new drills or switching up your focus.

5. **Stay Positive**: Focus on what you can control and the progress you're making, rather than dwelling on setbacks.

Overcoming Motivation Slumps

Even the most motivated gymnasts experience slumps. Here's how to get back on track:

- **Identify the Cause**: Are you feeling overwhelmed, bored, or discouraged? Understanding the reason behind your slump can help you address it.

- **Take a Break**: Sometimes, a short break can recharge your energy and enthusiasm.

- **Lean on Your Team**: Talk to your teammates or coach about how you're feeling. Their support can reignite your passion.

- **Revisit Your Why**: Reflect on why you started gymnastics and the goals you're working toward.

Real-Life Example: Rekindling Motivation

Maya, a gymnast in her third competitive season, found herself feeling unmotivated halfway through the year. Instead of giving up, she created a vision board filled with her goals, favorite gymnastics memories, and inspirational quotes. Seeing it every day reminded her of her love for the sport and helped her finish the season strong.

Activity: Motivation Booster

Try this activity to keep your motivation high:

1. Write down three reasons why you love gymnastics.

2. List two goals you want to achieve this season.

3. Create a mantra or motivational phrase to repeat to yourself during tough moments.

Keep these reminders in a place where you'll see them often, like your locker or gym bag.

The Power of Motivation

Motivation is what keeps you moving forward, even when the journey gets tough. By staying focused on your goals, finding inspiration in your teammates, and celebrating your progress, you can maintain your enthusiasm and achieve incredible things. Remember, every gymnast has moments of doubt, but it's your ability to keep going that defines your success.

Stay motivated, and you'll not only grow as a gymnast but also inspire those around you to reach new heights.

Chapter 16:
Building Leadership Skills

Leadership is about more than being in charge - it's about inspiring others, setting a positive example, and helping your team succeed. In gymnastics, every teammate has the opportunity to be a leader, whether by supporting others, showing dedication, or encouraging the team to stay united. Developing your leadership skills will not only strengthen your team but also prepare you for success in all areas of life.

What Makes a Great Leader?

Great leaders aren't born—they're made through practice, experience, and a commitment to growth. Key qualities of a strong leader include:

1. **Communication**: Clearly sharing thoughts, ideas, and feedback in a way that inspires and motivates.

2. **Empathy**: Understanding and valuing the feelings and perspectives of others.

3. **Integrity**: Leading with honesty, fairness, and respect for everyone.

4. **Resilience**: Staying calm and focused, even during challenging situations.

5. **Confidence**: Believing in yourself and your team while inspiring others to do the same.

Ways to Develop Leadership Skills

Here are practical steps to strengthen your leadership abilities:

1. **Lead by Example**: Show dedication, positivity, and respect in everything you do. Your actions set the tone for the team.

2. **Take Initiative**: Look for ways to help your teammates, organize activities, or solve problems without being asked.

3. **Listen Actively**: Pay attention to your teammates' thoughts and concerns and make them feel valued.

4. **Stay Positive**: Keep morale high by focusing on solutions instead of dwelling on problems.

5. **Encourage Collaboration**: Foster teamwork by involving everyone in decisions and ensuring all voices are heard.

Leading in Different Roles

Leadership in gymnastics isn't limited to captains or senior teammates. Here are ways to lead from any position:

- **As a New Teammate**: Bring fresh energy and enthusiasm to practice and routines.

- **As a Peer**: Support your teammates by offering encouragement and advice.

GYMNASTICS: How To Be the Best Teammate

- **As a Veteran**: Share your experience and mentor younger teammates to help them grow.

Real-Life Example: Leading Through Support

During a high-pressure meet, a gymnast named Ryan noticed his teammate struggling with nerves before her routine. Instead of focusing solely on his own performance, Ryan offered words of encouragement and helped her practice calming techniques. His leadership and support boosted her confidence, and she delivered a strong routine. Ryan's actions inspired the entire team to uplift one another.

Activity: Leadership Reflection

Take a moment to reflect on your leadership journey. Write down:

1. A time when you demonstrated leadership in gymnastics.
2. A leadership quality you'd like to develop further.
3. One action you can take to be a better leader for your team.

Share your reflections with a coach or teammate, and ask for their feedback on your leadership strengths and areas for growth.

The Impact of Leadership

Great leaders bring out the best in themselves and their teammates. By developing your leadership skills, you can inspire your team to work harder, stay united, and achieve incredible results. Remember, leadership is not about being perfect - it's about striving to make a positive impact every day.

Step into your role as a leader and watch how your team and personal growth soar to new heights.

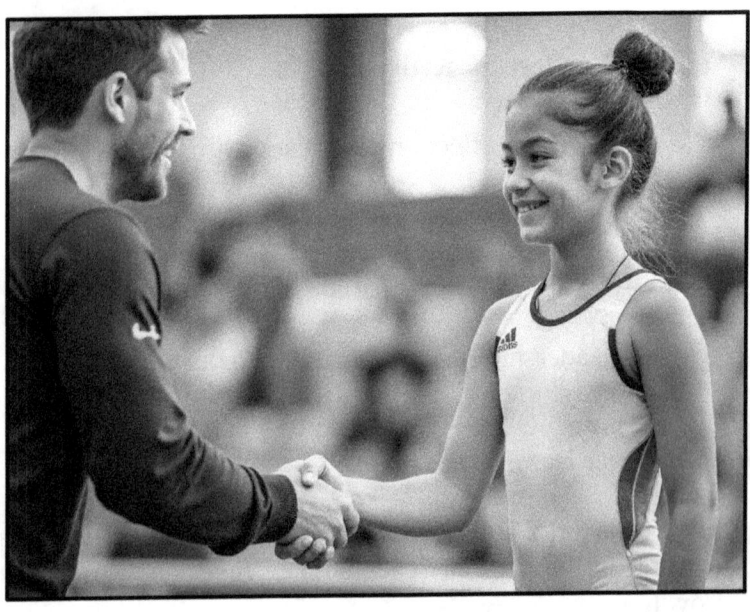

Chapter 17:
Being Prepared for Practice

Preparation is the key to a successful gymnastics practice. It sets the tone for your performance, helps you stay focused, and ensures that you get the most out of your time in the gym. By showing up prepared, you demonstrate your commitment to the sport and your team, setting yourself up for growth and success.

Why Preparation Matters

Being prepared for practice has many benefits:

1. **Maximize Learning**: When you come ready to practice, you can focus entirely on improving your skills.

2. **Prevents Injuries**: Proper preparation, like warming up and wearing the right gear, helps keep you safe.

3. **Shows Dedication**: Preparedness reflects your commitment to both your personal growth and your team.

4. **Boosts Confidence**: Knowing you're ready allows you to approach practice with a positive mindset.

How to Prepare for Practice

Here are some steps to ensure you're fully prepared for every practice session:

1. **Pack Your Gym Bag**: Make a checklist of essentials, including:
    - Leotards or practice attire
    - Water bottle
    - Healthy snacks
    - Grips, tape, and any other necessary equipment
    - Extra hair ties

2. **Arrive Early**: Give yourself time to settle in, warm up, and mentally prepare for the session.

3. **Eat Well**: Fuel your body with nutritious meals and snacks before practice to ensure you have the energy to perform your best.

4. **Warm Up Properly**: Spend time stretching and doing light cardio to prepare your muscles and prevent injuries.

5. **Set Goals**: Before practice, think about what you want to accomplish. Having specific goals helps you stay focused and motivated.

GYMNASTICS: How To Be the Best Teammate

Mental Preparation

Physical readiness is only part of the equation. Mental preparation is just as important. Here's how to get in the right mindset:

- **Visualize Success**: Picture yourself successfully completing skills and routines.

- **Stay Positive**: Focus on what you can control and approach practice with a growth mindset.

- **Clear Your Mind**: Leave distractions at the door and center your attention on the tasks ahead.

Common Preparation Pitfalls and How to Avoid Them

Even the best athletes can sometimes feel unprepared. Here are common pitfalls and tips for overcoming them:

1. **Forgetting Gear**: Double-check your bag before leaving for practice to avoid missing essential items.

2. **Rushing**: Plan ahead to ensure you have enough time to get to practice without stress.

3. **Skipping Warm-Ups**: Always prioritize warming up, even if you're short on time.

4. **Neglecting Rest**: Make sure you're getting enough sleep so you're alert and ready to perform.

Real-Life Example: The Power of Preparation

During a busy week of school and extracurricular activities, Sarah realized she hadn't been preparing for practice as well as she usually did. She forgot her grips one day and felt rushed another, which affected her performance. Determined to improve, she created a checklist and set a reminder to pack her bag the night before. With better preparation, Sarah noticed a huge improvement in her focus and performance.

Activity: Create Your Preparation Plan

Try this activity to make preparation a habit:

1. Write down everything you need to do to prepare for practice (e.g., packing your bag, eating a snack, setting goals).

2. Create a daily checklist and stick it somewhere visible, like your locker or bedroom door.

3. Reflect after practice on how being prepared helped you perform.

The Rewards of Being Prepared

When you show up to practice prepared, you're ready to give your best effort and make the most of your time in the gym. Preparation isn't just about having the right gear, it's about setting yourself up for success physically, mentally, and emotionally. By making preparation a priority, you

GYMNASTICS: How To Be the Best Teammate

demonstrate your dedication to gymnastics and your teammates, paving the way for continuous improvement and growth.

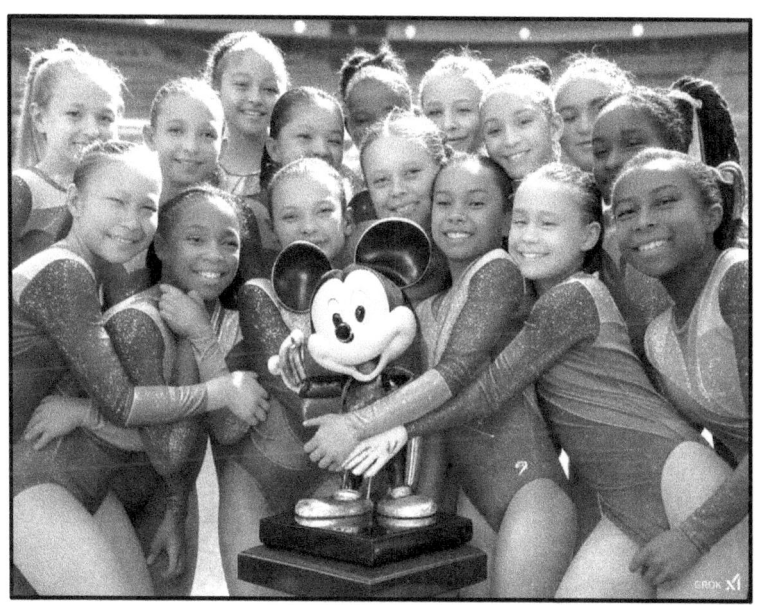

Chapter 18:
Responsibilities Beyond Training

For competitive gymnasts, training demands a level of dedication and discipline that rivals professional athletes. Hours in the gym perfecting routines, building strength, and maintaining flexibility can be grueling. But for young gymnasts, their responsibilities extend far beyond the gym. Balancing school, homework, chores, and family duties adds another layer of complexity to their already packed schedules. This chapter delves into how these young athletes navigate their multifaceted lives.

The Schoolwork Challenge

Education is a non-negotiable priority for every young gymnast, no matter how demanding their training schedule. Early morning practices or late-night gym sessions often leave little time for studying, but maintaining good grades is crucial. Time management becomes the key to success.

Gymnasts learn to maximize every moment of their day. They might review flashcards during car rides to the gym, squeeze in homework between training sessions, or wake up early to finish assignments. Many competitive gymnasts rely on planners to organize their tasks and deadlines, ensuring that school responsibilities don't fall through the cracks. Parents and coaches often step in to help, providing structure and encouragement while emphasizing the importance of balancing academics with athletic goals.

GYMNASTICS: How To Be the Best Teammate

Homework on the Go

Homework often travels with a gymnast - to meets, training camps, and even waiting rooms. Portable study tools like tablets, laptops, or old-fashioned notebooks are essential. Gymnasts develop a unique focus, able to block out distractions to complete assignments in unconventional environments. This adaptability not only benefits their academics but also builds resilience—a skill they carry into competitions.

Peer support also plays a role. Many gymnasts form study groups with teammates, tackling subjects together during breaks or downtime. This fosters a sense of camaraderie and shared responsibility, as they hold each other accountable for both athletic and academic performance.

Helping Out at Home

Even with their packed schedules, gymnasts are often expected to contribute at home. Simple chores like folding laundry, washing dishes, or tidying their rooms teach responsibility and provide a sense of normalcy. Some families implement chore schedules tailored to fit around training commitments, ensuring that the gymnast can participate without feeling overwhelmed.

Helping out at home is not just about the tasks themselves; it's also about maintaining family bonds. Sitting down for a family meal or pitching in during weekends reminds gymnasts that they are part of a team off the mat as well.

Parents often emphasize that teamwork at home mirrors the collaboration and mutual respect needed in the gym.

The Power of Routine

Successful gymnasts thrive on routine. A well-structured day allows them to tackle their responsibilities without becoming overwhelmed. For instance, a typical weekday might look like this:

- **6:15 AM**: Wake up, eat breakfast, and review school notes.

- **7:30 AM**: Attend school.

- **3:30 PM**: Head to the gym for training.

- **7:30 PM**: Return home, eat dinner, and start homework.

- **9:00 PM**: Wind down with light stretching or reading before bed.

This disciplined schedule not only ensures that tasks are completed but also teaches valuable time-management skills that will serve gymnasts well into adulthood.

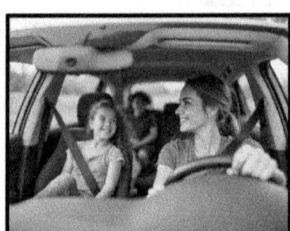
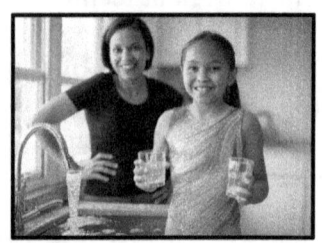

GYMNASTICS: How To Be the Best Teammate

Coping with Stress

Juggling multiple responsibilities can be stressful, even for the most organized gymnast. To manage this, many turn to strategies like mindfulness exercises, journaling, or talking with mentors. Coaches and parents play a crucial role, offering support and understanding during particularly demanding periods, such as competition season or exam weeks.

Encouraging open communication is key. Gymnasts who feel comfortable expressing their challenges are better equipped to find solutions, whether it's adjusting their training schedule temporarily or seeking academic help.

Lessons Beyond the Gym

The demands of being a competitive gymnast extend far beyond the physical challenges of the sport. Balancing training with school, homework, and family responsibilities teaches invaluable life skills like discipline, time management, and resilience. These young athletes learn to prioritize, adapt, and persevere, setting them up for success not just in gymnastics but in every aspect of their lives.

For a gymnast, the balance beam isn't just a piece of equipment in the gym – it's a metaphor for their daily life. Keeping steady, maintaining focus, and finding balance are the keys to thriving in their dual roles as students and athletes. And when they do, the rewards are as fulfilling as nailing a perfect routine.

Conclusion:

Congratulations! By exploring the chapters of this book, you've taken a deep dive into what it means to be the best teammate in gymnastics. From building trust and celebrating successes to staying motivated and being prepared, you've learned valuable lessons that will not only strengthen your team but also help you grow as an individual.

The Core Values of a Great Teammate

Throughout this journey, we've emphasized key qualities that define the ultimate teammate:

1. **Trust and Respect**: Building strong relationships through honesty and kindness.

2. **Responsibility and Preparation**: Showing up ready to give your best effort.

3. **Support and Sportsmanship**: Uplifting your teammates and competitors with humility and integrity.

4. **Resilience and Motivation**: Facing challenges with a positive mindset and determination.

5. **Leadership and Teamwork**: Inspiring others and working together toward shared goals.

GYMNASTICS: How To Be the Best Teammate

These values don't just make you a better gymnast - they make you a better person.

The Ripple Effect of Your Actions

Being a great teammate has a ripple effect that extends beyond the gym. Your dedication, positivity, and support inspire others to strive for their best, creating a stronger, more unified team. As your actions influence those around you, you become a role model for future gymnasts who look up to you.

Your Gymnastics Journey

Gymnastics is about more than mastering skills and winning medals – it about the relationships you build, the lessons you learn, and the person you become along the way. By embracing the principles in this book, you're not just setting yourself up for success in the sport—you're preparing for success in life.

Remember, the journey to becoming the best teammate ever is ongoing. There's always room to grow, learn, and make a difference.

A Final Challenge

As you continue your gymnastics journey, I challenge you to:

1. Reflect on what you've learned in this book and how you can apply it to your daily life.

2. Set one new goal to become an even better teammate.

3. Share your knowledge and experiences with others, helping them grow alongside you.

A Note of Encouragement

Being the best teammate ever isn't about being perfect - it's about showing up every day with a positive attitude, a willingness to learn, and a commitment to supporting those around you. You have the power to make a lasting impact on your team, your sport, and beyond. Keep striving, keep growing, and keep being an amazing teammate.

Thank you for taking this journey. The gym floor is yours! Go make a difference!

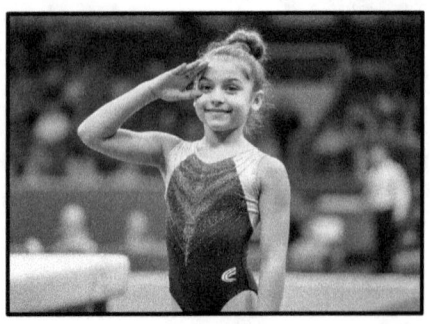

GYMNASTICS: How To Be the Best Teammate

Journaling Ideas to De-Stress and Feel Happy

Included in your journaling should be some of these items.

1. Things you enjoy (for breakfast, relaxation, school, etc.)

2. Fun things that you'd like to change

3. New things you'd like to try

4. List of things you're grateful for

5. Things you can see from where you're sitting

6. Bucket list of places you'd like to visit

Here's an outline for what should be included in a young gymnast's daily journal:

Date: Write the day's date to keep track of progress

Goals for Today:

List 1-3 specific goals for today's session.

- ➤ Examples might include:
1. Perfect my back walkover.
2. Increase the number of push-ups by 5.
3. Work on balance on the beam for 10 minutes.

Warm-Up:

• Quick notes on what warm-up exercises were done to prepare the body for training.

Training Activities:

• Skills Practiced: Briefly note the gymnastics skills or routines worked on.

• Sets/Reps/Time: If applicable, how many times or for how long each skill was practiced.

Challenges:

• Mention any difficulties encountered during the session, like trouble with a particular move or feeling less energetic.

Accomplishments:

• Highlight what went well or any small victories, even if it's just feeling more confident with a move.

Coach's Feedback:

• If available, write down any advice or feedback from the coach.

Conditioning:

• Note any strength, flexibility, or endurance exercises done, e.g., number of pull-ups or time spent stretching.

Cool Down:

• Brief mention of the cool-down routine to signify the end of the session.

Physical Feelings:

• How did the body feel? Any soreness, pains, or areas that feel stronger?

Emotional State:

• How did you feel today? Motivated, frustrated, happy, etc.

Notes/Reflections:

• A space for any additional thoughts, what was learned, or what to focus on next time.

Tomorrow's Focus:

• Optionally, a quick note on what to concentrate on in the next session.

This outline helps in systematically recording daily progress, reflecting on performance, and setting clear, achievable goals, which are crucial for growth in gymnastics.

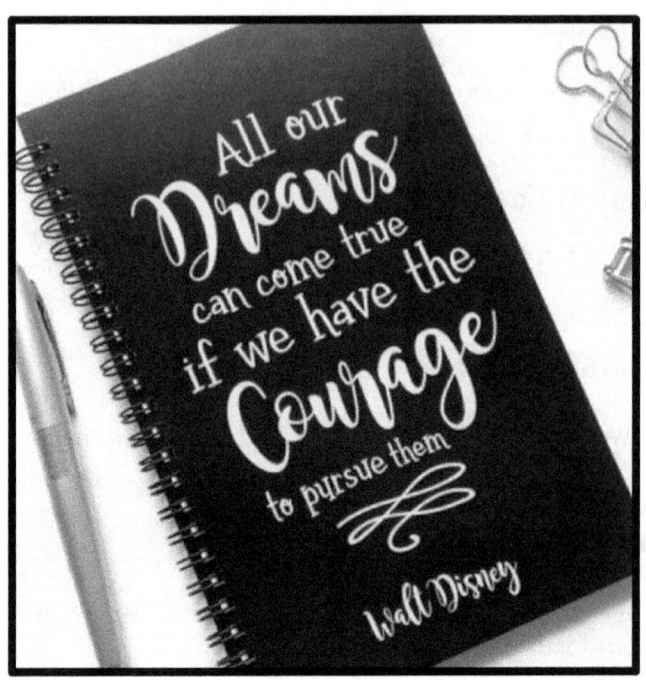

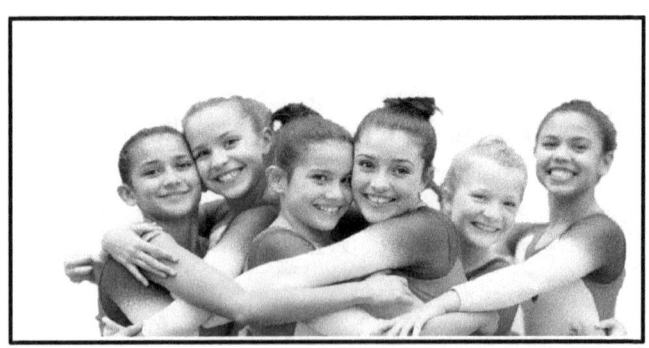

About the Author

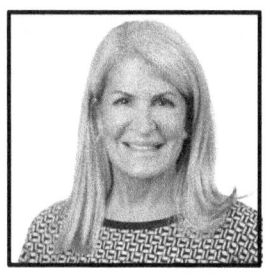

Rita Brown has established herself as an iconic figure in the world of gymnastics. Over her illustrious career, she has coached more than forty athletes to the USA National Team and guided them to win over 100 national and international medals. A two-time Olympic coach, Rita's expertise has propelled gymnasts to compete at the highest levels, including the Olympic Games in 1988, 1992, 1996, and 2004, as well as the 1997 World Championships. Her passion for the sport transcends competition, evident in her founding of Brown's Gymnastics Training Centers, which grew to seven locations across the United States, and her contributions to gymnastics education through her partnerships with USA Gymnastics University.

Rita's influence extends to the literary arena with her numerous publications, including *Gymnastics: Your Best Meet Ever!* and several *Gymnastics Coaches Certification Manuals*. These works are indispensable resources for coaches and athletes, emphasizing safe training practices, building self-confidence, and fostering the self-esteem of young gymnasts. Her books not only offer technical guidance but also provide a roadmap for achieving success in both gymnastics and life, solidifying her as a thought leader in the field.

In addition to her coaching and literary accomplishments, Rita has made significant contributions to gymnastics safety and education. As an expert witness in gymnastics-related incidents and the founder of GYMCERT.COM, an online program for coach certification and safety awareness, she has worked tirelessly to improve standards within the sport. Her dedication to gymnastics extends further, having served two terms on the Board of the USA National Gymnastics Foundation, showcasing her commitment to sport's long-term growth and sustainability.

Rita Brown's extraordinary career reflects her multifaceted talents as a coach, author, entrepreneur, and advocate. Her lasting impact on gymnastics continues to inspire athletes, coaches, and fans worldwide, ensuring her legacy as a true innovator and mentor in the sport.

GYMNASTICS: How To Be the Best Teammate

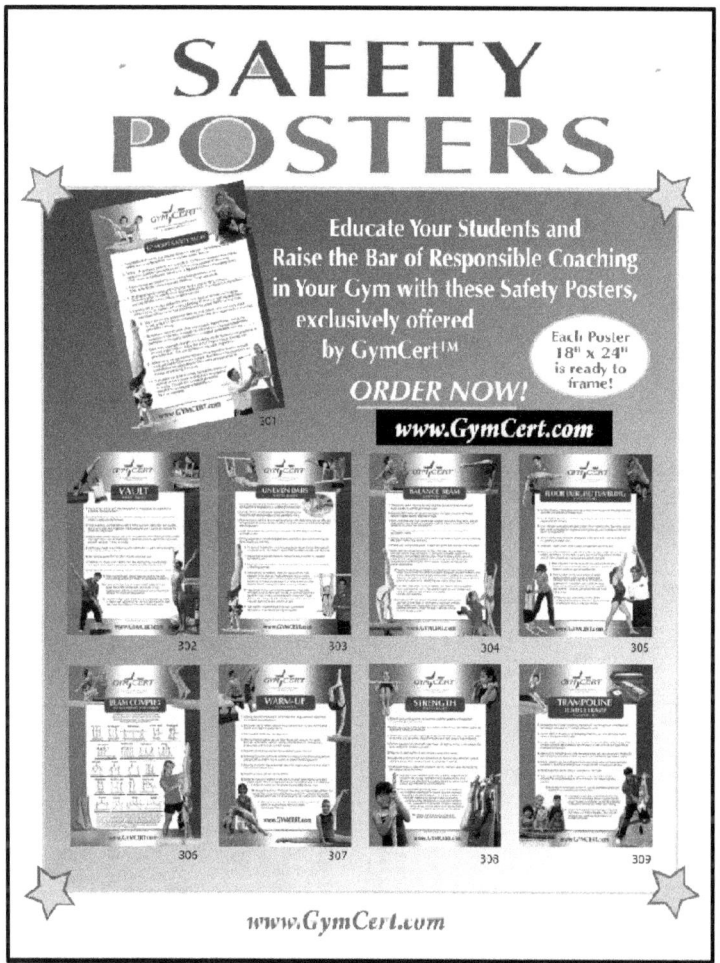

Rita Brown

NOTES

www.ingramcontent.com/pod-product-compliance
Lightning Source LLC
LaVergne TN
LVHW051845080426
835512LV00018B/3079

9781938975011